THE SACRED STRUGGLE

THE
SACRED
STRUGGLE

Jewish Responses to Trauma

Edited by Rabbi Lindsey Danziger
and Rabbi Benjamin David

Foreword by Rabbi Charlie Cytron-Walker

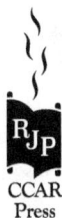

RJ**P**
CCAR
Press

Reform Judaism Publishing, a division of CCAR Press
CENTRAL CONFERENCE OF AMERICAN RABBIS
5785 NEW YORK 2025

Unless otherwise noted, Torah translations are from *The Torah: A Modern Commentary, Revised Edition*, ed. W. Gunther Plaut (CCAR Press, 2006), and other Biblical translations are from *The JPS Tanakh: Gender-Sensitive Edition* (Jewish Publication Society, 2023).

Published by Reform Judaism Publishing, a division of CCAR Press
Central Conference of American Rabbis
355 Lexington Avenue, New York, NY 10017
(212) 972-3636 | info@ccarpress.org | www.ccarpress.org

LIBRARY OF CONGRESS CATALOGING-IN-PUBLICATION DATA
Names: Danziger, Lindsey, 1986, editor. | David, Benjamin, 1977, editor. |
  Cytron-Walker, Charlie, 1975, writer of foreword.
Title: The sacred struggle : Jewish responses to trauma / edited by Rabbi
  Lindsey Danziger and Rabbi Benjamin David; foreword by Rabbi Charlie
  Cytron-Walker.
Other titles: Jewish responses to trauma
Description: New York: Reform Judaism Publishing, a division of CCAR
  press, 5785/2025. | Series: CCAR challenge and change series |
  Summary: "Addressing trauma, resilience, and post-traumatic growth
  through a Jewish lens, this volume provides respite, relief, and the
  realization that trauma is universal and healing is possible."
  —Provided by publisher.
Identifiers: LCCN 2024060262 (print) | LCCN 2024060263 (ebook) | ISBN
  9780881236620 (trade paperback) | ISBN 9780881236637 (ebook)
Subjects: LCSH: Psychic trauma. | Jews—Mental health.
Classification: LCC RC451.5.J4 S33 2025 (print) | LCC RC451.5.J4 (ebook)
  | DDC 296.3/8—dc23/eng/20250218
LC record available at https://lccn.loc.gov/2024060262
LC ebook record available at https://lccn.loc.gov/2024060263

Text design and typography by Scott-Martin Kosofsky
  at The Philidor Company, Rhinebeck, NY. www.philidor.com

Cover design by Barbara Leff.

Printed in the U.S.A.

10 9 8 7 6 5 4 3 2 1

Contents

Foreword

Rabbi Charlie Cytron-Walker

I refer to it as "The Incident."

The use of euphemisms was one of many things I learned in Jerusalem during the first year of rabbinical school at Hebrew Union College–Jewish Institute of Religion.

That year (2001–2), we experienced ten major terrorist attacks in Jerusalem and over thirty throughout Israel. We were encouraged to avoid going out on Saturday nights and avoid crowds in general. Then, on March 9, 2002, just shy of 10:30 p.m., a terrorist went to Café Moment and blew himself up, murdering eleven civilians in the process. Rabbis and HUC-JIR students were on their way to the café. Some of my classmates lived right across the street. The attack on Café Moment was a traumatic end to our formal year of education.

Throughout the year, we never called it the "Second Intifada" or acknowledged it as a "war." Instead, taking our cues from the Israelis of all backgrounds with whom we interacted every day, we referred to it as *hamatzav*, "the situation."

So, after three of my congregants and I survived an almost eleven-hour hostage situation on January 15, 2022, at Congregation Beth Israel (CBI) in Colleyville, Texas, it felt natural to refer to it in a similar way, to search for language to provide some distance from an event I will always carry with me.

The Incident began like any other Shabbat morning at the tail end of the pandemic. We were having services in person, but most people were participating online. I arrived before 9:30 a.m. I was setting up the projectors, loading the slides, and turning on the sound system. At a small congregation, these tasks are all part of the rabbi's role.

But this morning, unexpectedly, there was a visitor at our door. He asked if we had a night shelter. It was cold for Texas—in the thirties—and he looked like he had spent the night on the street. I saw someone who needed to warm up. I opened the locked door and asked him if he wanted some coffee. He asked if we had any tea. We chatted as the water was heating, and I didn't register any concern.

I made sure the visitor was situated and then returned to my preparations for that morning's service. The service began; a dozen people joined online, three congregants attended in person, and our visitor remained in the back of the small sanctuary next to the kitchen.

During the *Amidah*, the central portion of our worship service that begins with the prayer *Avot*, remembering our ancestors, and ends with *Shalom*, praying for peace, I was turned toward Jerusalem with my back to the congregation. I thought I heard the click of a gun—a sound that I remembered from a visit to a gun range. It could have been the metal roof of the building or the ice machine or any of the other common noises our building would make. I was leading *G'vurot*, the prayer praising God's power. I turned my head right away and didn't see anything amiss, but I was worried enough that during silent prayer I walked back to inform the visitor that he didn't have to stay for the whole service. That's when he pulled the gun on me.

Immediately he started shouting. "I love death more than you love life," he yelled over and over, throughout the day. He said he had bombs. He told us to call 911 and clear the area near the synagogue so no "innocent" people would be harmed. Then he asked to speak with Rabbi Angela Buchdahl of Central Synagogue in New York City. My heart sank. In that moment, I knew that he actually believed all the lies and conspiracy theories about Jews: Jews control the government, the banks, the media—Jews control everything. He traveled from England all the way to our tiny congregation in Colleyville, Texas, with the hope that he could kidnap Jews and get a convicted terrorist out of jail.

In those initial moments I felt an absurd mixture of emotions: Fear to have a gun pointed at us. Terror for my congregants. Concern for my family and the rest of the congregation. And gratitude that he didn't want to kill as many Jews as possible—he "only" wanted to take us hostage. Over the course of the day, we learned that the congregation was relatively close to the federal prison where the jailed terrorist was being held, although I never focused on why The Incident was happening.

There was a man with a gun in my synagogue, and my attention was consumed by the reality of the moment and doing anything I could to help us get out of there alive.

In the afternoon, over four hours into "The Incident," after extensive work by the FBI negotiation team and some smart thinking on the part of one of my congregants, the gunman released Larry, an older gentleman. That was an incredible relief, but it was far from the end of our ordeal.

As evening fell, the gunman became more agitated. He was yelling more and demanding more from the FBI negotiator. He became infuriated because he was not getting what he wanted. I let my fear get the best of me then, breaking down and trying to appeal to his humanity. That did not work. He saw my emotion as a weakness. Going forward, I did everything I could to rein in my emotions and focus on what I could do in the moment.

Shortly afterward, the gunman told the FBI negotiator that he was going to have us kneel down and kill us one at a time until he got what he wanted. He had been so angry, but after he hung up, he suddenly became very calm—which was absolutely terrifying. That's when he asked for a drink.

I walked into the kitchen; he could see me the whole time. When I opened the fridge, he asked for soda. So I poured him a cup, gave it to him, and then went back to where I had been seated.

He then started to preach to us. He told us again how he had been compassionate, but now would no longer be compassionate. It was like he was working himself up. As he was doing this, I noticed that he had one hand over the top of the gun, not on the trigger. The other hand was holding the cup of soda. I realized that this was one of the best opportunities that we'd had all day.

I told Jeff and Shane (the other two hostages) to run, and then I picked up a chair and threw it at the gunman. We were out the door before a shot could be fired. About thirty seconds later, after we were all safely behind an armored vehicle, we heard the explosion of the FBI breaching the building. And then we heard gunfire. The gunman was killed. None of the hostages or any law enforcement personnel were physically injured. This was a moment of shock, profound relief, and gratitude.

I couldn't stop shaking from the adrenaline. We were all amazed and incredibly thankful to be alive.

The Incident was certainly traumatic for those of us who were held hostage. It was also traumatic for the CBI community and the Colleyville community. It was traumatic for so many in the Jewish community—in the United States, in Israel, and around the world—who were glued to their phones and televisions and were symbolically with us in the synagogue that day. For many, the communal trauma and fear after the Tree of Life, Poway, Colleyville, and October 7 continue to this day.

In the aftermath, I was surrounded by family, inundated with media requests, and still needed to be the rabbi of a congregation that had just gone through a horrible ordeal. It was impossible not to be fully cognizant that it could have been so much worse. I also had to take care of myself in that moment.

More than anything else, I needed to see people, hug people, and simply be with people. That's why we held a healing service on Monday evening, just two days after The Incident. That evening, I shared a message of gratitude for all the support we received and the fact that we didn't have to say *Kaddish*. I acknowledged the trauma that was experienced, the healing that was needed, and the importance of receiving love and empathy after such a challenging ordeal. While I suspect that my congregation needed it, I *know* that I needed it. And, indeed, it was incredibly healing for us all.

We couldn't use our building for three months while repairs were made. Our local Jewish Family Service truly cared for our community, including leading special sessions for our youth. I took advantage of the mental health resources that were available. We received an unbelievable amount of love and support from the Jewish people, from our Colleyville community, from Israel, and from all over the world. In the days and weeks following The Incident, we needed every bit of the overwhelming kindness we received.

We also leaned into Jewish tradition to create moments of comfort for both the wider congregation and those of us who had been hostages. When the four of us recited *Birkat HaGomeil*—a prayer to acknowledge a near-death experience—it brought comfort. When we were finally able to return to the synagogue, we held a private event where we marched our Torah scrolls down the street and back into our building. By doing so, we reclaimed the sacredness of our Jewish home. And the next day, when we welcomed the whole Colleyville community back into the building, we did our best to express gratitude for all who had embraced and uplifted us. There were countless conversations, moments of kindness, and great care given to security issues. And healing, of course, takes time. For some, that healing is still ongoing in many critical ways.

What happened in Colleyville offers some important lessons, many of which you will also read about throughout this volume. Trauma is never easy. Everyone experiences trauma differently. Following trauma, everyone needs love and support, and what that means for each person will vary considerably. Trauma is overwhelming when trying to cope as an individual. Going through a more public trauma adds layers of complexity.

Practically, it was invaluable that we hired an incredible media consultant, who protected us from reporters and helped us approach the media strategically. Personally, I had to get used to people meeting me and bursting into tears. It didn't happen every day, but it happened often enough. My understanding is that when people met me or saw me for the first time afterward, they started reliving all the emotions they felt in that moment, which made it easy to be able to offer a hug and offer them support in that moment.

I feel blessed to have been able to walk away from that day. Any time we can walk away from a trauma is a blessing, even if the trauma stays with us. While a *r'fuah sh'leimah* (complete healing) may not be possible, some form of healing or coping is often attainable. Trauma disrupts us. It doesn't end us. As hard as it can sometimes be to find it, there is a way forward. That is why this volume, with all of the challenges and difficulties presented, is ultimately about hope.

Trauma may shatter us. It doesn't have to end us. Whenever we finish reading a book of the Torah, we recite, "*Chazak, chazak, v'nitchazeik.* Be strong, be strong, and let us strengthen one another." In our struggles, we may not feel any strength. With help and support, we can be strengthened. There is a way forward. I pray that this volume can be a source of strength for you.

Acknowledgments

Rabbi Lindsey Danziger
and Rabbi Benjamin David

Tractate *Taanit* of the Babylonian Talmud teaches that scholars sharpen other scholars (7a). Throughout this process we learned so much about the trauma of our people. We sharpened each other as our understanding of loss, pain, and the strength of the human spirit became sharper. This book came about following our meeting at a CCAR convention many years ago, when we connected over our personal experience with cancer as young rabbis. We bonded over the unique questions that cancer raised for clergy members who deal each day in faith, Torah, and Jewish community. More than anything, we considered how our trauma had changed us, strengthened us and reshaped our understanding of ourselves and our Judaism. Over the course of this process, we learned from each other, lifted each other up, agonized together, and remained steadfast in creating an anthology that would resonate with others, provide direction, and grant a measure of hope to those in need of it.

This book would not be possible without the expert guidance of the CCAR and CCAR Press, including Rabbi Hara Person for her leadership and guidance, Rafael Chaiken for his attention to detail and thoughtfulness, Rabbi Annie Villarreal-Belford for her endless patience, keen eye, and great expertise. She was a constant source of support and help. We would also like to thank Deborah Smilow and Raquel Fairweather-Gallie for their behind-the-scenes work and Debra Hirsch Corman, Michelle Kwitkin, Barbara Leff, and Scott-Martin Kosofsky for their contributions, which refined and elevated the book.

Thank you to our editorial committee for their time and attention to this important project. Every contributor to the book offered significant time, vulnerability, and insight. We are so grateful. We would like to acknowledge Rabbi Charlie Cytron-Walker for writing the foreword. Both his harrowing experience and his newfound sense of perspective set the perfect tone for this work. Thank you as well to Dr. Betsy Stone for her consultation and wisdom as we sought to define trauma in Jewish terms and think carefully about the goals of the book.

Thank you to our many teachers along the way and the communities we have the great pleasure of working with. You must take credit for this book as well. Finally, thank you to our families and communities for their never-ending support and love.

Introduction

RABBI BENJAMIN DAVID

AFTER AARON's two sons perish in a priestly ritual gone horribly wrong, Aaron is famously silent (Leviticus 10:1–3). The dramatic scene in the Book of Leviticus at once feels completely unrelatable and entirely familiar. We are often without words when overwhelmed by emotion. Aaron will join a long list of Biblical figures who are stunned outright by tragedy. In Genesis alone, we read of Noah, who watches a world drown (Genesis 6); Abraham, who witnesses Sodom and Gomorrah go up in smoke (Genesis 18–19); and Joseph, who is cast out by his own brothers (Genesis 37). We read of a burgeoning Israelite community that, starving, seeks out sustenance in the land of Egypt, a place totally foreign to them, only to suffer four hundred years of slavery (Genesis 46; Exodus 1–2). Much of the Torah is built around the Children of Israel, who endure the harsh climes of the wilderness as they trek to the Promised Land. Moses himself will experience the heartbreak of never entering the Land of Israel; he is granted only the consolation of seeing it from afar (Deuteronomy 34:4). His inevitable feelings of disappointment are easily understood by anyone who has ever come up short or been left wondering what might have been. Despite these trials, our Biblical ancestors managed to hold onto their faith—a faith that evolved as they did. During and following episodes of deep distress, they maintained a sense of connection to their God and their people that was genuine and deep-rooted.

Later portions of the Hebrew Bible also present a suffering people who, through it all, held onto their sense of belief and heritage. The Psalmist recounts how, exiled from Israel, wallowing in Babylon, "there we sat; sobbed, as well, when Zion came to mind" (Psalm 137:1). Even amid such dire moments, our Biblical ancestors found a way to "give thanks to [God] with all my heart—before magistrates mighty as gods, it is to You I will sing. I will fall prostrate before Your holy place and I will give praise to Your name, for Your covenantal love and Your truth" (Psalm 138:1–2).

Job, altogether beleaguered by loss and tragedy, still manages to proclaim to the Eternal One, "I know that You can do everything, that nothing You propose is impossible for You" (Job 42:1). Such sagas of exile and steadfast devotion have stayed with and within the Jewish people. Returning to faith is a motif that of course transcends Bible and midrash, assuming a very real place in modern Jewish history as well. Perhaps this communal muscle of faith was—even ironically— strengthened most by our parents and grandparents as they fled their European homes and communities mere decades ago. Indeed, who can count the remarkable tales of belief that emerged from the Holocaust? As so many abandoned religion during that most gruesome chapter in our story, so did many grow stronger in their connection to Jewish life when surrounded by death. The stories read like legends: Shabbat prayers uttered quietly in concentration camp barracks, marking Simchat Torah against all odds, somehow lighting a makeshift menorah during Chanukah. Moreover, so many survivors of the Holocaust returned to synagogue, observance, and worship as they constructed their lives anew. How did they do it? Why did they do it? Elie Wiesel and others have argued that in the aftermath of the Shoah, the return to Jewish life came precisely because we need words: Once the shocked silence dissipates, we long to give shape and voice to our wounds and experiences. In *The Six Days of Destruction*, Wiesel notes, "We need altars and rituals and worship. . . . There comes a time, as it came to Job after his long and brooding silence, when one has to stand up and cry out. That cry is prayer. It addresses God, and it addresses humanity."[1] This speaks to a type of faith that is part of our healing and goes beyond platitudes, taking us to a place that is outright transformative.

We twenty-first-century Jews are of course well versed in trauma. With the lessons of the Holocaust still ringing in our ears, we have encountered no shortage of stinging antisemitism and hatefulness in our own day. Whether in Charlottesville, Pittsburg, Poway, Jersey City, or Monsey, the relentless attack on Jews and Judaism has shaken all of us. We have grieved together and in time adjusted to a "new normal" in which antisemitism is less an abnormality and more a reality to be wary of every day. We do so amid a post-9/11 world that feels at times desperately unstable: a world where school shootings happen with regularity; where racism, homophobia, transphobia, and xenophobia are rampant; where bullying and cyberbullying plague our children; and where the natural world is under attack by forces that range from small to existential. We feel in our heart for Israel—all the more so since October 7, 2023—too often maligned or outright denigrated by the international community, even as we mark the highly imperfect record of our beloved Israel. Terror within and outside of Israel has wounded our Israeli family for generations and, by extension, all of us.

How do we not turn to anger? Or, better yet, how do we cling to a Judaism of relevance and hope even in our anger and frustration? How do we maintain a relationship with a benevolent God in illness, in mourning, in dire sadness and frustration? Is it acceptable for a long-standing relationship with Judaism and the Divine to change following a period of distress? What does it mean to reevaluate one's sense of Jewish heritage from a hospital room or a place of quiet grief? This book will explore these important questions, and more.

To be clear, by choosing to title this book *The Sacred Struggle*, we are not saying we believe nor will we argue that everything happens for a reason, nor offer up a type of theology that is clichéd or unhelpful. Rather, this title affirms that the act of struggle itself can become part of our sacred life journeys. By bringing together writers who have experienced profound hardship and been changed by that hardship, this book aims to shed light on what it means to hold onto Judaism during life challenges and give permission to earnestly evolve in our relationship to faith.

Rabbi Danziger and I both experienced cancer early in our rabbinic career. We were both young parents at the time, with young kids. We each learned a lot about trauma—trauma of the body and the spirit, and how trauma affects a family and community. Cancer is what brought us together, and our journey since has led to the creation of this book. We have both thought at significant length about the ways in which trauma can be life altering, both in ways that are negative and in ways that are surprisingly positive. We have both thought extensively about the pains we each carry and that our people carry. We have wondered together about themes of healing and change, both as human beings and as rabbis. This book comes therefore from both a deeply personal and professional viewpoint.

The Sacred Struggle begins with a useful definition of trauma from Dr. Betsy Stone before exploring the theme of trauma from a textual angle: What do our earliest sources teach us about Jewish responses to trauma? The chapters explore Biblical, Rabbinic, and contemporary approaches to trauma. We then examine different areas of potential trauma: the trauma of acute and chronic illness and how physical challenges impact our emotional and spiritual well-being; the trauma that can result from being marginalized because of race, gender, ability, or illness; the impact of personal and communal violence, from the streets of Memphis to the school halls of Parkland, from terror events to sexual assault; the trauma of natural disasters and the all-too-familiar trauma of pandemics; the trauma that can occur when one is part of a larger community that may be toxic, unhealthy, or simply not present; and finally, the trauma of family loss, which manifests as divorce, infertility, stillbirth, and death of loved ones. Of course, just because we chose to group certain experiences of trauma does not mean that we are equating the experiences; every trauma is different, as is each of these beautiful, harrowing chapters. Indeed, each chapter goes to a highly vulnerable place; there is great honesty in this book. We believe that within these pages there is something for everyone. We have all lost. We have all been hurt. We can likely all find value in exploring the tools that these brave authors present us.

Here is a taste of what the following pages will offer readers: Rabbi Lawrence A. Hoffman, PhD, explores the ways liturgy can support us in the face of traumatic events. Rabbi Dalia Marx, PhD, takes us through Israeli poetry and song created in response to the horrific events of October 7. Rabbi Daniel B. Gropper shares with us his near-death experience and the lessons he learned. Rabbi Iah Pillsbury shares her deeply moving and troubling story of abuse and the connections she made to the Biblical figure of Esther. Rabbi Joel Mosbacher takes us through his painful and very personal understanding of gun violence. Rabbi Rex D. Perlmeter, LSW, and Rabbi Susan Talve both share with us what they learned as a result of what many might consider the ultimate loss, the loss of a child. These pages are indeed more than heart-wrenching. They are more than inspiring, for they offer us an array of resources as we each carry our respective pains and burdens. These accounts are not merely to be read, therefore, but seen as guideposts for any of us attempting to seek out those Jewish ideas that can help us in the aftermath of crisis and incidents of trauma.

This book does not reflect every traumatic experience—we could not be 100 percent comprehensive. There are so many historical traumas, so many natural disasters, so many personal stories and experiences every single person endures; to capture them all is simply not possible. Still, we hope you find yourself and your own story broadly reflected in the experiences we share. Our intent was to offer a resource and point of connection for readers who may have undergone similar traumas or experiences, but we recognize that everyone reacts to these stories differently. To that end, we encourage you to be careful while reading this book, as some chapters will be difficult to read and may speak closely to your own trauma. The majority of chapters contain resources, especially Jewish resources, and stories of how individuals have navigated their own trauma; still, we encourage readers to take care of themselves and actively seek out the support they need. Consult your own rabbi for support, or seek out a trauma-informed therapist for deeper work. There are a number of additional organizations with online and in-person resources that can offer unique support depending on what you might be facing; these include National Alliance on Mental Illness (NAMI), Alcoholics Anonymous, the American Cancer Society, and many others. If you are feeling suicidal, call 988 and seek emergency support. You do not need to suffer alone.

May this book offer you some guidance, some help, and some comfort. May it remind us of the strength we all hold within and the awesome fortitude that runs through our Jewish story.

NOTE
1. Elie Wiesel and Albert H. Friedlander, *The Six Days of Destruction: Meditations Toward Hope* (Pergamon Press by arrangement with Elie Wiesel and the CCAR, 1988).

Defining Trauma
What It Is, What It Does, and How It Changes Us

BETSY STONE, PHD

WHAT IS TRAUMA? A book focusing on the experience of trauma *should* have a definition. But definitions, by their very nature, are imperfect. Any definition will bias the reader toward a particular point of view. Can a trauma be ultimately positive? Are there "happy" traumas? Do we define trauma by the event or by its impact? Are there events that are universally traumatic? And how idiosyncratic is trauma anyway?

While this collection will explore different experiences of trauma, we must understand that trauma is defined by the one experiencing it—not by some objective, external evaluation. What is traumatic for me may be a typical life event for you. Trauma is experienced by a person (possibly within a group of people), and that person determines the impact of a situation—not by calmly evaluating it, but in their reactions, their kishkes.

While we clearly live in traumatic times, we do not all respond to traumatic circumstances in the same way.

Early in COVID, I led a Zoom meeting on trauma. I used a definition that is freely available on the internet—that "trauma is the response to a deeply distressing or disturbing event that overwhelms an individual"—and described the aspects of trauma—an inability to cope or feel the full range of emotions, feelings of helplessness, diminished sense of self—inherent in that definition.[1] One person, a man who lived in a war zone and worked with refugees, took exception. He said, "That's not trauma. That's simply how I live." For him, calling COVID a trauma was simplistic. He reminded me how trauma is actually deeply personal. Our understanding of trauma is influenced by our culture and our personal experience.

So how do we begin to define trauma? The American Psychological Association defines it as follows: "Trauma is an emotional response to a terrible event like an accident, rape, or natural disaster."[2] Even this one-sentence definition raises questions. What is a terrible event? Does the event have to be "terrible" for it to produce trauma? Are all emotional responses evidence of trauma? Does trauma come from a real event, or can it appear in reaction to an anticipated event, which might not even occur?

Yet, this definition is also clarifying. Trauma is *not* the event. Trauma is the emotional response to the event. Trauma lives in the person, not in some objective evaluation. I get to define that which is traumatic for me.

This idea is important. A traumatized person does not need the agreement of others to experience trauma. As with fear and grief, it is common for people describing their own emotional responses to receive reactions that diminish or deny their reality. "It's not that bad" or "You're overreacting" are messages designed to *comfort* the listener, but all they ultimately do is teach the listener that the person sharing these words cannot be trusted with feelings. We cannot offer comfort if we do not respect the individual emotional power of loss and pain.

So, we have clarified one important aspect of trauma: It is the emotional response. Are there other aspects?

Trauma (like most of our experiences) happens in our brains. We may experience trauma in our bodies, as with physical assault, but part of the experience is always in our brains. Our brains house our emotional response to traumatic events. And it's not happening in our rational brains, our thinking brains. Rather, it's happening in a more primitive part of our brains, the limbic system.

The limbic system is part of our brain's survival mechanism. It is always scanning for danger and reacts with fear, rage, or anger. It is a control system for dealing with danger and emotionally difficult experiences. It is where we begin to store emotional memories. It helps us pay attention, when we can. And it only seems to have "language" that is associated with noise—laughter, growling, and crying—rather than words. This is why we cannot use logic or even words to process in the limbic system.

In order to understand or interpret events, we need our frontal lobes. This area, in the front of our brains, is where we manage language. Here, we make meaning, engage in voluntary activities like walking or eating, pay attention, and develop complex ideas. Our frontal lobes can communicate with our limbic system, but this communication is less effective when we are aroused or fearful.

When trauma occurs, the limbic system is immediately aroused. Our brains flood with cortisol, a stress hormone, which allows us to escape from real or perceived danger. Our thinking brain in the frontal lobes takes a back seat to our reactive brain in the limbic system, which pushes us to respond with one of three built-in defense mechanisms: flight, fight, or freeze.

Over time, we can begin to process trauma in our frontal lobes, using language to understand experiences. However, we store our memories of trauma through the limbic system, so trauma is stored without verbal understanding. It's stored as a physical experience, not a cognitive one. Our bodies remember trauma by smell, sound, kinesthetic memory. And our brains store trauma for our entire lives.

What this means for us is that every new trauma pulls up every old trauma. People with a long history of trauma are therefore more sensitive to subsequent trauma. We do not "get over" trauma; we manage it. We never become untraumatized. We integrate the trauma into our life view. Trauma is much like grief in this way. For some of us, the way we integrate trauma might look like post-traumatic stress disorder (PTSD). For others, there are paths of growth that result from trauma. This is called post-traumatic growth.

This information extends our definition: Trauma is an individual emotional response *and* we do not get over it.

Another important facet about trauma is that it is not always bad stuff that causes trauma, but it is always disruptive stuff. For instance, the birth or adoption of a first child, which changes my relationship to myself in the world and to the world, can be traumatic—even though the birth or adoption is a positive event. Research tells us that birth or adoption can be even as traumatic as the death of a parent. Trauma— from a positive or negative event—changes how I understand myself.

Trauma can be personal, and it can be communal. Communal

trauma changes the trajectory of history, while personal trauma changes the trajectory of a life. We might posit, for example, that the communal trauma of the Holocaust was essential in convincing the United Nations to support the establishment of the State of Israel. Or we might suggest that the collective reaction to the COVID pandemic changed the outcome of the 2020 election.

Personal trauma can change the trajectory of a life. The March for Our Lives community arose out of the personal traumas of students who survived the mass shooting at Parkland High School. Mothers Against Drunk Driving, or MADD, arose from the tragedies of children killed by inebriated drivers. In both cases, the experiences of individuals changed the focus of their lives. We might also see this with less dramatic life events such as infertility, depression, or educational challenges.

Trauma—even communal trauma—can be intensely isolating. While we might assume that others experience trauma in the same ways we do, often they do not. For example, siblings may react differently to the death of a parent. These differences can make us feel that something is wrong with us or others around us; they can make us feel alone. People may say, "I understand how you feel," but they do not. My feelings are my feelings. They are fluid, idiosyncratic, and unpredictable.

So we respond differently to different communal traumas. Let's think about three examples: 9/11, COVID, and October 7.

The terrorist attacks on 9/11 resulted in a sudden, intense, communal trauma. It united people across the globe. Part of our response to 9/11 was to give blood, but another part was to take revenge. As individuals we tried to help. As a community, we fought back (even if the fight was wrongly directed). Ultimately, 9/11 was unifying.

COVID-19 was a gradual, chronic trauma that was both communal and personal. We lost friends and family members, and we lost trust in institutions. We began to doubt the government and its instructions. We saw everyone we encountered as potentially lethal. Both because it was long and because it was isolating, the impact of COVID-19 is harder to pin down. We lost trust in the decisions of other people, whether they were pro- or anti-mask, pro- or anti-vaccine. Many pundits and politicians focused naturally on loss of life, yet we must also attend to the very real loss of social skills we saw in both children and adults. These "soft" skills are more difficult to measure but may impact societies for decades. The lingering sense that other people are potentially deadly impacts our social relationships to this day.

The events of October 7 were a tribal trauma. For many Diaspora Jews, October 7 revealed our deep sense of commitment to other Jews. It was not simply a national trauma, but a trauma that united Jews around the world. Jews who had no deep feelings about Israel suddenly felt connected. Jewish pride rose. And antisemitism exploded. Our sense of safety was challenged everywhere. Many of us felt more deeply Jewish, more afraid, and more proud. Others tried to hide their Judaism, removing mezuzot from external doors, taking off Jewish jewelry, or covering *kippot* with baseball caps. We also felt isolated from those who did not seem to understand the depth of our grief. One rabbi said to me, "I'm not interested in interfaith dialogue with people who don't care about me." The feeling of being in this particular tribe and *not* in the general population was scary, sad, and deep.

This adds to our definition. Trauma is personal and idiosyncratic. We do not get over it. We only heal forward. And trauma can impact individuals, communities, and tribes.

Some communal traumas are widespread enough to define a generation. Vietnam altered the relationship between the government and the governed for baby boomers and beyond. It is conceivable that the 2023 war in Israel will significantly shape and define Israelis and Diaspora Jews going forward. In both these cases, citizens began to question the role and effectiveness of their government. Moreover, in both these cases, one did not have to be physically present to experience trauma.

This is called secondary or referred trauma. People in helping professions—clergy, medical personnel, therapists—are familiar with the distress that can come from hearing the stories of people directly traumatized. Again, remember that distress rises to the level of trauma in a personal, idiosyncratic way. As a therapist, I may be able to hear some stories of trauma and not experience them personally. Others will touch me too deeply—either because of similarities to my own lived experience or because I am simply vulnerable at that moment.

We helpers may make light of secondary trauma. We may feel that we are not "entitled" to hurt as badly as we do. We say to ourselves, "After all, it didn't happen to me." Denying the impact of the traumatic stories we hear from others doesn't make them less potent. It simply makes us ashamed for our deep feelings. While there is no doubt that I must control my emotional reactions while listening to a painful story, that does not mean I must deny its impact on me. We need to find ways to be present for others *and* create time and space to process the impact of their stories. Simply naming their impact will help. Helpers who experience secondary trauma also need to recognize and accept that they, in turn, may need help absorbing the stories they hear. Clergy, like others in helping professions, are exposed to trauma frequently. And as helping professionals, clergy must remain aware of their personal response to others' trauma as a clue that they are getting overwhelmed. And for anyone who experiences trauma, it is important to refocus and give yourself recovery time. Sometimes it's important to seek help yourself—from a trusted colleague, friend, or therapist. Clergy, helping professionals, and every other person who experiences trauma needs to give themselves permission to address their own pain.

This is an important point about any kind of negative emotion. Naming it helps. As soon as I can identify what I'm feeling, my relationship to that emotion changes. We know that named negative emotions decrease and named positive emotions grow. The pain I experience when I hear an awful story is real, and naming (and accepting) that makes it more manageable. I need to name my feeling, and I need to accept that I have the right to that feeling. The goal is *not* to be above my feelings; it is to accept and know my feelings.

Complications may arise when our secondary and primary trauma overlap. In COVID, the aftermath of October 7, or in natural disasters, we heard stories and witnessed pain that was both external and internal.

This, too, expands our definition of trauma. Trauma is a personal emotional response resulting from individual, tribal, communal, or secondary events and whose impact is lifelong.

So how do we heal? As I mentioned above, when we speak about trauma, we may use words like "recovery" and phrases such as "back to normal." These approaches are simply not helpful, because—according to our definition—trauma is not something we recover from. We cannot recover from trauma, but we *can* heal. It is important to remember, though, that healing from trauma is not a return to a previous state. Rather, healing is an integration of the traumatic experience into a new worldview. Healing from trauma is post-traumatic growth—integrating the trauma with new understandings of ourselves in the world. Healing is forward motion, not backward.

Post-traumatic growth involves six types of positive psychological changes that are the result of struggle with trauma and/or challenging situations. No one does all of them; remember, the goal is not to complete growth, but to *incorporate* growth. The six areas are as follows:

1. New understanding of personal strengths.
2. Increased spiritual growth (which should be distinguished from religious or ritual growth, although they may overlap).
3. Increased creativity.
4. Deepened relationships and the shedding of unimportant relationships.
5. Deepened values and a stronger sense of possibility.
6. Greater appreciation of life; increased gratitude.

Post-traumatic growth may involve any one or more of these arenas of growth. The presence of post-traumatic growth does not preclude PTSD and the ongoing impact of trauma. In fact, humans do not resolve trauma; we learn to manage it. Like grief, there are times when trauma manages us and other times when we manage trauma. The goal in living with trauma is to integrate traumatic experiences into our understanding of ourdelves and the world.

Some people respond to personal trauma by digging deeply into the source of that trauma. People who are sexually assaulted may become counselors. Families who have lost a child to cancer may lead groups for other parents. These are examples of post-traumatic growth; we can use our pain to support other people.

Ultimately, trauma—like fear and grief—changes the ways our brains function. We may be hyper-alert or slowed down. We may feel fuzzy and unfocused. We may be locked into a permanent stress response. We can't accelerate the ways we process these intense experiences, but we can forgive ourselves for the struggle they create. As we work to help and support others, we also seek our own help and support, so we can create and navigate those critical paths from trauma to growth.

NOTE
1. "What Is Trauma?," Integrated Listening, posted September 13, 2018, https://integratedlistening.com/blog/what-is-trauma/.
2. "Trauma" American Psychological Association, https://www.apa.org/topics/trauma.

PART ONE

Jewish Textual Foundations for Understanding Trauma

1

Job's Traumatic Breach

ADRIANE LEVEEN, PHD

H E IS A SIMPLE, pious man blessed with a predictable cycle of ordinary days and celebratory festivals.[1] He has ten children, who gather together while he offers sacrifices in each of their names. His life is full. Suddenly, those days and that predictability are torn asunder. His life becomes a nightmare as he sets out to understand how and why he has been so tragically struck. This is the story of the Biblical character Job, considered among the righteous, whose trauma unfolds in the Biblical book named after him. As Job comes to realize that God is the source of his suffering, Job experiences a breach in his belief in God's loving-kindness, fairness, and justice. He is shattered and traumatized. Yet by story's end, Job has found a way to recover. His is a story in which many readers over the centuries have found solace and guidance. Perhaps we can too.

Psychiatrist David Lindy, with whom I studied the Book of Job, works with people suffering from trauma. He links Job's trauma to betrayal. Lindy argues that after experiencing God as a caring parent, it makes sense that Job would suffer terribly once tossed aside. God does exactly that in the prologue to the Book of Job (chapters 1 and 2) by allowing Job to suffer at the hands of a heavenly figure, the Adversary.[2] God permits the Adversary to strip Job of his wealth, property, and most tragically, his children. Why? God has agreed to a wager with the Adversary to disprove their claim that Job would curse God if everything was taken away from him. To prove the Adversary wrong and reassure the Divine Self, God bets on Job's loyalty and unwavering faith. God's only condition: The Adversary must spare Job's life.

Job is wholly unaware of the wager but does accurately place the ultimate responsibility with God. After all, God's need to prove Job's loyalty leads God to grant the Adversary horrific power, allowing Job to be abused while taking no action. It is hardly a stretch to understand that Job would perceive God's treatment of him as mystifying and even abusive. Soon enough, for the first time, Job comes to question the ways of God.

As the narrative unfolds, Job relinquishes his former expectation of God acting as a caring parent. Job begins to protest his treatment and searches for divine answers to the injustice done to him. Struck by unexpected and unimaginable events, Job moves through stages of heartbreaking grief and fury. Instead of waiting for divine justification, Job discovers what he needs to say to God. Once Job finds his voice and speaks truthfully about God's behavior, his trauma subsides and his recovery slowly begins. He is no longer the God-fearing man of the book's opening, yet he stays in relationship with God. Job also grows in a self-compassion that allows him to honor his own integrity, even if grief remains. In what follows, I trace certain moments in Job's story that allow him to return to the land of the living.

Struck by Tragedy

In the prologue, God permits the Adversary to go about destroying everything precious to Job. Job responds in act and word:

> Then Job arose, tore his robe, cut off his hair, and threw himself
> on the ground and worshiped. He said, "Naked came I out of my
> mother's womb, and naked shall I return there; God has given,
> God has taken away; blessed be God's name." (Job 1:20–21)[3]

The description captures Job's grief, yet, as we shall see, this is only his first response and is based on Job's instinctual piety toward God. His words capture God's attention, who reproaches the Adversary for inflicting Job *chinam*, "gratuitously," or "for no good reason" (2:3). Martin Buber notes the significance of the word *chinam*: "Here God's acts are questioned more critically than in any of Job's accusations, because here we are informed of the true motive, which is one *not* befitting to the deity."[4] Nonetheless, God allows the Adversary to continue their torments, and they next inflict Job with boils. We hear nothing more from God until chapter 38.

In his second response, Job continues to assume that God is the originator of these acts. "Should we accept only good from God and not accept evil?" (Job 2:10). Job adds a crucial word to his outburst, "evil." That is new. It is a sign that he is beginning to question his beliefs. As he mourns, Job acknowledges that God has sent evil his way.

At that moment three companions who live nearby hear of Job's woes and join him in silence for seven days (Job 2:11–13). Rabbi Mychal Springer points out that their initial actions provide a helpful model for a comforter: Show up. Be silent. Be present.

Job's Despair

Their silence does not last. Soon enough, Job breaks his in a bitter, devastating torrent of words, not against God but against himself. Job objects to being alive. This is psychologically astute on the part of the Biblical writer. Those who suffer trauma may blame themselves in self-loathing. Job expresses his own self-loathing in 3:1–6:

> Afterward, Job began to speak and cursed the day of his birth.
> Job spoke up and said:
> Perish the day on which I was born,
> And the night it was announced,
> "A male has been conceived!"
> May that day be darkness;
> May God above have no concern for it;
> May light not shine on it;
> May darkness and deep gloom reclaim it;
> May a pall lie over it;
> May what blackens the day terrify it.
> May obscurity carry off that night;
> May it not be counted among the days of the year;
> May it not appear in any of its months.

The first two verses emphasize four ways of speaking in the Hebrew, drawing our attention to the role of lamenting in trauma. Scholars Manfred Oeming and Konrad Schmid suggest that Job "must spit it out and work through his pain."[5] Job has no idea why this has happened or who precisely is behind this traumatic upheaval. He does not curse God, but does curse the day he came into the world. Articulating the extent of his angst and suffering allows Job to begin the hard work of reckoning with what has happened.

Job's wish to "perish" guides verse 3. "Born" and "conceived" are. mentioned in reverse order, as if by going back in time Job could blot out his very conception.[6] He wishes that he had never been brought into the cycle of time. The descriptive language he uses in verse 4 culminates in a darkness that utterly engulfs and blocks out light. This is a poetry of despair and of nonbeing.

You Must Deserve This Suffering

Job pours out his anguish to his increasingly uncomfortable and unsympathetic companions. Their responses to Job's suffering escalate as they listen to him question God's ways. Job is as articulate and honest as he can be. They see it differently and, forgetting their role as comforters, respond in anger. Springer suggests that they can't help themselves. But their harsh words, based on their understanding of tradition, greatly increase Job's pain. They are certain that God inflicts tragedy only on those who deserve it. Job must have sinned, says one, even if he doesn't know the reason. Another, oblivious to the terrible loss of the children, suggests that suffering is good for Job and will heal him. When their words of reproof fail to deter Job, they loudly remind him that he is obligated to submit to divine discipline and cease complaining.

The reader knows that the companions are terribly wrong in justifying God because we witnessed the wager God makes with the Adversary. Job's companions, however, are ignorant of God's motives. Their dogmatic reliance on cause and effect leaves them blind to the reality of their friend's pain and his character. They exacerbate the trauma afflicted on him by God and the Adversary. Simply put, they blame the victim. Their behavior warns us that when facing a traumatized friend, it is best to check our assumptions, temper our responses, and be attentive and silent.

Job Seeks God

Job becomes increasingly provoked by the companions' words. In response to their mistaken cliches, he gains clarity and realizes that his suffering is undeserved. He ceases to blame himself. Knowing how he has conducted his life, he insists on his innocence. He becomes his own advocate, turning his attention to the reality of divine injustice. Job finds his courage and his voice, demanding a day in court with God:

> I say to God, "Do not condemn me;
> Let me know what You charge me with.
> Does it benefit You to defraud,
> To despise the toil of Your hands,
> While smiling on the counsel of the wicked? (Job 10:2–3)

Job realizes that to believe in divine justice, cause and effect, sin and punishment, means to be blind to what actually takes place in the world. Trouble falls indiscriminately on the good and the bad, including Job.

God Appears Out of the Storm

Whatever move Job takes away from trauma to ordinary existence will not bring back his children. The grief of those losses will remain for the rest of his life. But turning away from self-blame to scrutinize God does allow Job the capacity to continue to live. As it happens, Job's defiant stance toward God triggers God's reappearance in chapter 38. This is not the day in court sought by Job, nor does God directly respond to his request. Nonetheless, God chooses to be present. God shares with Job knowledge of God and the natural world of which Job was unaware. God weaves together a poetry of the constellations in the heavens, the surging of the sea, and the slow movement of dawn's light along the sand. God shows Job an array of wild animals and birds that exist for their own sake, not for human beings. Job is invited to fully perceive God's created world at its most expansive.

God boasts of a most threatening creature, the Leviathan. Whether as mythic god of the sea or a very aggressive crocodile, Leviathan strikes terror in the human heart:

> See, any hope [of capturing] it must be disappointed;
> One is prostrated by the very sight of it.
> There is no one so fierce as to rouse it;
> Who then can stand up to Me? (Job 41:1–2)

Job, mere human as he is, doesn't stand a chance. God seems intent on putting Job in his place. The natural world does not circulate around him. Nor is it about justice, which Job has come to understand as a solely human concern. Nature is about cycles of seasons, destruction, and regrowth.[7] Yet God's reappearance is paradoxical. While Job is not the center of God's Creation, God cares enough to continue the conversation. God has shown up. This is a crucial step in Job's recovery.

Rabbi Jeremy Kalmanofsky describes the effect of knowing that we, like Job, are minor players, not just in our vast world, but in the vast universe we can now observe thanks to the James Webb Space Telescope. Kalmanofsky conveys his awe toward an ever-expanding universe: "The cosmos is so vast it silences the mind. . . . Theologically, I must conclude that all this cannot be about us. . . . On earth and in worlds beyond, across sextillions of stars and in subatomic spaces, God is the Name of Existence—its breathing and its beating heart."[8] Kalmanofsky cites Maimonides, who reminds us that "the best worship is to fall silent before the reality surpassing understanding."[9] Kalmanofsky's description of God—vis-à-vis the creatures on one tiny planet in the universe—aptly and beautifully fits the tenor of God's message to Job. Silence is the appropriate response, first to Job's suffering and now as Job stands silently in awe before a God he will never fully understand. Answers cannot be found; this is perhaps unsatisfactory, except to the degree that it seems authentic. Mystery remains. Nonetheless, Job has experienced something of the Divine Self. God is not changing the subject but is expanding Job's awareness.

Job's Compassion for Humanity

How does Job respond? Job is equivocal.

> Job said in reply to God:
> I know that You can do everything,
> That nothing You propose is impossible for You. (Job 42:1–2)

Job concedes that God is powerful, but he already knew that after his children were killed. He knew that with his very body as he lay writhing in pain. God's power is not an answer to what Job seeks.

In a footnote to the introduction of his remarkable translation of Job, Edward Greenstein explains Job's reference to himself in 42:6 as "dust and ashes." He suggests the Biblical phrase refers to wretched humanity.[10] No longer blaming himself, Job does not acquiesce entirely to God. Job does remain in relationship with God. Simultaneously, he experiences compassion toward a humanity in which suffering is widespread. He is not alone.

God's Presence

God's last words are a crucial final step on Job's path to recovery. As Job's companions reappear, God rebukes one named Eliphaz:

> After God had spoken these words to Job, God said to Eliphaz the Temanite, "I am incensed at you and your two friends, for you have not spoken the truth about Me as did My servant Job . . . . Since you have not spoken the truth about Me as did My servant Job." (Job 42:7a, 42:8b)

There is no typo here. God twice points out that Job has spoken the truth. As put by David Lindy, God may not be what Job, or his companions, had expected. Yet the Biblical writer vindicates Job as God concedes the justice of Job's case. Transformed by what has happened to him while retaining his integrity, Job has returned to himself.

Job's Path Back

Those who attend to Job's steps on his long journey toward recovery might discover in Job a helpful exemplar. He begins by articulating a fervent wish for nonexistence. His honest, even brutal, expression of feeling sets the stage, waking him to the new emotional state he must face. Job quickly experiences an anger triggered by his friends' misguided rebukes that helps him to clarify his blamelessness and fuels his search for truth. Finding his voice and his agency leads Job to compassion for himself and for others who have also suffered. In recognizing the vulnerability of being human, a vulnerability that he shares with others, Job is no longer alone. God's concession to Job at the very end is also significant and offers a model for us, mere mortals that we are. If we can be present with those who have suffered from trauma, listening carefully and acknowledging their experience, they in turn may find comfort in the telling. Together we can celebrate their truth of themselves in its fullness.

NOTES

1. I taught some of these ideas during a webinar on June 2–3, 2021, titled "Moral Injury and Soul Repair: A Jewish Perspective" as part of *A Conference for Clergy and Mental Health and Other Helping Professionals*. I thank Rabbi Nancy Wiener for an invitation to present Job at that conference. As I wrote this essay, I was blessed to have personal conversations with Rabbi Lisa Goldstein, Rabbi Mychal Springer, and Dr. David Lindy. I am grateful to them for their insights and their friendship.

2. In his brilliant 2019 translation and commentary, Edward L. Greenstein describes the Biblical role of the Adversary: "The Satan's role is to accuse and prosecute people for their transgressions. The title is derived from a term meaning 'obstruction' (Numbers 22:32) or 'opposition' (I Samuel 29:4). The Satan seeks to trip up human beings and then report on their missteps; but he is also the contrarian who contradicts the opinions of God" (*Job: A New Translation* [Yale University Press, 2019], 5n20).

3. Translations of the Book of Job in this chapter are from *The JPS Tanakh: Gender Sensitive Edition* (Jewish Publication Society, 2023), found on Sefaria (sefaria.org).

4. Martin Buber, *The Prophetic Faith*, trans. Carlyle Witton-Davies (Harper and Row, 1960), 190. I came to Buber's thinking on Job via Steven Kepnes, "Rereading Job as Textual Theodicy," in *Suffering Religion*, ed. Robert Gibbs and Elliot R. Wolfson (Routledge, 2002).

5. Manfred Oeming and Konrad Schmid, *Job's Journey: Stations of Suffering* (Eisenbrauns, 2015), 28.

6. Robert Alter, *The Art of Biblical Poetry* (Basic Books, 1985), 98.

7. As put to me by Rabbi Lisa Goldstein.

8. Rabbi Jeremy Kalmanofsky, "Cosmic Theology and Earthly Religion," in *Jewish Theology in Our Time*, ed. Rabbi Elliot J. Cosgrove (Jewish Lights, 2010), 23–25.

9. *Guide for the Perplexed* I:59, cited in Kalmanofsky, "Cosmic Theology," 28.

10. Greenstein, *Job*, 185n9.

2

Talmudic Responses to Trauma

RABBI DVORA E. WEISBERG, PHD

> The Sages were at the wedding of Mar, son of Ravina. They turned to Rav Hamnuna Zuti saying, "Sing something for us." He responded, "Woe to us, for we will die; woe to us, for we will die." They asked, "How shall we respond?" He replied, "Where is the Torah and the mitzvah that will protect us?"
>
> —*Babylonian Talmud*, B'rachot 31a[1]

THIS STORY tells us that Rav Hamnuna, even on the festive occasion of a wedding feast, was focused on the inevitability of death. Although he proposes a response to that awareness—seeking refuge in the study of Torah and the observance of commandments—one imagines this provided very little comfort to him or his colleagues. This exchange follows two stories about rabbis who, while hosting their sons' weddings, broke valuable vessels because they thought that their guests were rejoicing too much. Collectively, these three stories suggest that the Rabbis were uncomfortable with what they perceived as unbridled joy, even on a special occasion. In the words of Rabbi Shimon bar Yochai, "A person is forbidden to fill their mouth with laughter in the here-and-now"; such joy will only be permissible when God redeems Israel (Babylonian Talmud, *B'rachot* 31a). Our Rabbis were, it seems, incapable of sustained happiness, perhaps as a result of what we might describe today as generational trauma.

What was the source of this trauma? We don't know much about what individual rabbis experienced in their personal lives, but their words indicate that they were traumatized by the destruction of Jerusalem in 70 CE, had lost any hope of national self-determination in the wake of two failed revolts against Rome, and most of all, possessed a profound sense of alienation from God. These feelings are captured in the response they suggest to a would-be convert: "Why do you want to convert? Don't you know that [the people] Israel, at the present time, is broken, harried, driven, and tossed about, and trouble has come upon them?" (Babylonian Talmud, *Y'vamot* 47a). Even as the Babylonian Talmud exhorts us to direct our prayers toward God, Rabbi Elazar asserts that "from the day the Temple was destroyed, the gates of prayer were locked. . . . An iron wall separated Israel from their Father in heaven" (Babylonian Talmud, *B'rachot* 32b).

Trauma can be defined as an experience that is frightening or painful or as the lasting impact of that experience on a person, sometimes over a long period. One of the challenges of exploring trauma in Rabbinic stories is that these stories are snapshots of a moment in time. We read about a rabbi having a disturbing experience, but we don't know what their life was like before that experience or how it impacted the rest of their life. We do not hear stories told by the individuals themselves, and we cannot ask questions that might help us consider the lasting impact of trauma. Rabbinic stories are shaped by the editors of the collections in which they are found, and these editors or redactors may have lived hundreds of years after the rabbis in the stories they are relating. The redactors shaped them for particular contexts and to support their own understanding of the significance of the stories' events. We might feel that Rabbi Shimon bar Yochai's fury at seeing people engaged in ordinary activities was the result of spending twelve years hiding in a cave (Babylonian Talmud, *Shabbat* 33b) or that the trauma of being publicly humiliated and shunned by colleagues led Rabbi Eliezer ben Hyrcanus to pour out his heart in prayer, leading to the death of Rabban Gamliel (Babylonian Talmud, *Bava M'tzia* 59b), but we don't know enough from these stories to diagnose these rabbis.

One example of a story that might be best understood through the lens of a traumatic event features Nachum Ish Gam Zo:

> They said of Nachum Ish Gam Zo that both his eyes were blind, both his hands and feet were crippled, and his entire body was covered in boils. His home was in disrepair, and the legs of his bed had been set in bowls of water so ants would not crawl on him. His students wanted to remove his bed and then remove the other furnishings. He said, "My sons, first remove everything else, and then remove my bed; you can be certain as long as I am in the house, it will not collapse." They removed everything else

and then removed his bed, and then the house collapsed. They said, "Rabbi, since you are an utterly righteous person, why has all this befallen you?"

He said to them, "My sons, I caused [my ailments] myself. Once I was on my way to my father-in-law's, and I had three laden donkeys with me; one carried food, one drink, and one various types of delicacies. A poor person came and stood in my path, saying to me, "Rabbi, sustain me." I said, "Wait while I unload the donkey." Before I could unload the donkey, the poor person died. I threw myself on him and said, "May my eyes, which took no pity on your eyes, be blinded. May my hands, which took no pity on your hands, be crippled. May my feet, which took no pity on your feet, be crippled." I didn't calm down until I said, "May my entire body be afflicted with boils." They said, "Woe to us that we see you like this." He said, "Woe to me if you did not see me like this." (Babylonian Talmud, *Taanit* 21a)

Nachum attributes his physical suffering to his failure to respond quickly enough to save the poor man's life. But his reaction seems extreme and uncalled for. How could he have known how urgent the man's need was? How could he have helped him without opening the saddlebags and taking out food to give to the starving man? And even if Nachum is convinced that he is responsible for the man's death, is his embrace of ongoing suffering the appropriate expiation for his act of involuntary manslaughter?

The editor of our *sugya* (section) has no overt comment on this story. Instead, the *sugya* continues with a question, "And why did they call him Nachum 'Ish Gam Zo' [a man who says "this too"]? Because every time something happened to him, he would say, 'This too is for the good.'" Then the *sugya* offers the following example of Nachum's positive outlook on life:

Once, the Jews needed to send a gift to Caesar. They said, "Who will go? Let Nachum Ish Gam Zo go, since he is accustomed to miracles." They sent with him a bag filled with precious stones and pearls. He went and spent the night in an inn. That night, the people at the inn got up, emptied his bag, and filled it with dirt. The next day when he saw it, he said, "This too is for the good."[2] When he arrived at his destination, they opened the bag and saw that it was full of dirt. The king wanted to kill all of them, saying, "The Jews are mocking me." He said, "This too is for the good." Elijah came, appearing to him as one of them. He said, "Perhaps this dirt is the dirt of their father Abraham. When he tossed the dirt, it became swords, and the clods became arrows." There was a country that they had been unable to conquer; they checked out the dirt and conquered the country. They took Nachum into the treasury and filled his bag with precious stones and pearls and sent him off with great honor. He returned and stayed at the same inn. They said, "What had you brought with you that caused them to honor you so much?" He said, "What I took from here is what I brought there." They razed their inn and took the material to the king's house. They said to him, "The dirt that he brought was ours." They checked it out and found it was not so, and they executed the people from the inn.[3]

In this story, Nachum finds himself in peril. He has come to Caesar's court with a bag of dirt, rather than the bag of precious stones he intended to present on behalf of his community. Not only is Nachum in danger of losing his life, but the entire Jewish community is at risk. What is Nachum's response? "This too is for the good." Nachum survives because a miracle occurs. Elijah appears and suggests to Caesar that the apparently worthless—and insulting—gift has magical properties; it can produce weaponry that ensures victory. Instead of being executed, Nachum is rewarded and sent home in honor.

The story closes by relating how the inhabitants of the inn, who robbed Nachum and sent him off to almost certain death, got their comeuppance. Eager to capitalize on what appears to be a market for dirt, they offer the authorities more dirt. However, they are not Nachum Ish Gam Zo; no miracle is performed on their behalf, and they are executed. In the version of the story in *Sanhedrin* and in manuscript editions of *Taanit*[4] we are unsure whether Nachum knew that he had been robbed and was now carrying dirt to Caesar. Only in the Vilna edition does Nachum open the bag before arriving at his destination. Regardless of whether and when Nachum realizes that he has been set up, his exchange with the inhabitants of the inn on his return trip, intentionally or inadvertently, leads to their deaths. Unlike the previous story with the poor man, there is no indication that Nachum feels any vindication or responsibility for these deaths.

The order of these stories allows us to consider how the events of the second story might shed light on why, in the first story, Nachum accepts—and even embraces—his suffering. Earlier in life, when he was still well enough to undertake a journey to Caesar, Nachum narrowly escaped death. At the time, he denied that he was afraid or upset, and insisted, "This too is for the good." But perhaps the Babylonian Talmud is hinting at the long-term effect of this near-death experience. If Nachum was traumatized by his encounters with the thieves and the Roman government, might he have lost his rosy view of the world? Might his later insistence that he was responsible for the death of the poor man in the road be delayed guilt, the response of a man traumatized by the sense that he had caused the death of the inhabitants of the inn and had endangered the lives of his fellow Jews through his naivete? Does the structure suggest that a traumatic experience can shape a person's behavior and self-understanding for years after the experience?

The Rabbinic response to personal and generational trauma took several forms. Rabbis minimized or embraced sadness and pain, spoke about the value of suffering as an aid to atonement, or saw the present pain of the Jewish people as a precursor to national restoration. We learn that the third-century sage Rabbi Yochanan came to visit his student Rabbi Elazar and found him weeping. Yochanan mused over the source of Elazar's tears, wondering aloud if Elazar was sad that he had not studied even more Torah or about his lack of wealth. Perhaps, Yochanan said, you are sad about children, presumably a reference to Elazar's lack of children or the death of some of his children. Well, said Yochanan, holding up an object, "this is the bone of my tenth son." Elazar told his teacher that he was crying because "'of the beauty [of Rabbi Yochanan] that will [someday] be swallowed by the earth.' Rabbi Yochanan responded, 'That is certainly a reason to weep,' and they both wept." After weeping with his ailing student, Yochanan asks, "Are your sufferings dear to you?" and Elazar replies, "Neither they nor their reward." After this negative reply, Yochanan stretches out his hand and raises his student up (Babylonian Talmud, *B'rachot* 5b). Rabbi Yochanan carried with him a physical reminder of his tragic loss—the death of multiple children—as well as the awareness of his own mortality, but he also sought to alleviate the suffering of others.

Rabbinic stories that expose the trauma caused by the destruction of the Temple and the loss of autonomy also speak to the dangers of being overly caught up or immersed in one's pain. A story is told of an encounter between Rabbi Y'hoshua and people who responded to the destruction by denying themselves meat and wine:

> Our Rabbis taught: When the Second Temple was destroyed, ascetics abounded in Israel. They would not eat meat, nor would they drink wine. Rabbi Y'hoshua engaged them in conversation. He said, "My children, why do you not eat meat? Why do you not drink wine?" They responded, "Should we eat meat, when once it was offered on the altar and now it can no longer be offered? Shall we drink wine, when once it was offered as a libation on the altar and now it can no longer be offered?" He said, "If so, we should no longer eat bread, for the meal-offerings have ceased. It is possible to survive on fruit . . . but we should not eat fruit, for the first fruits can no longer be offered. It is possible to survive on other fruits. . . . We should not drink water, for the water libation can no longer be poured out [on the festival of Sukkot]."
> [The ascetics] were silent. [Rabbi Y'hoshua] said, "My children, come and I shall teach you. Not to mourn at all is impossible, for the evil decree has been carried out. To mourn too much is also impossible, for it is forbidden to set a stricture on a community if the stricture is too hard to bear. . . . Rather, the Sages teach: A man plasters his house but leaves a small portion unplastered. . . . A man prepares a meal but leaves out a small portion. . . . A woman puts on her ornaments but leaves off a small item." (Babylonian Talmud, *Bava Batra* 60b)

Rabbi Y'hoshua's advice to the ascetics is telling. He acknowledges that they have experienced a tragedy that they cannot forget, an event that may mark the rest of their lives. He doesn't tell them to "get over it" or to ignore the experience and focus solely on the future. Rather, he affirms the need to acknowledge and even create visual reminders of their traumatic experience. At the same time, he cautions them not to embrace their trauma to the exclusion of living.

In closing, I want to consider a story from *Avot D'Rabbi Natan*.

Rabban Yochanan ben Zakkai and Rabbi Y'hoshua are walking near Jerusalem and see the Temple ruins. Y'hoshua is distressed over the loss of the Temple, the place where Jews atoned for their sins through sacrifices. Yochanan consoles him, saying, "Do not grieve. We have another way to atone, and what is it? Deeds of loving-kindness [*g'milut chasadim*], as it is said, 'For I desire loving-kindness, not sacrifice' (Hosea 6:6)" (*Avot D'Rabbi Natan* 4). We cannot deny the impact of traumatic events on our lives. Our tradition teaches that we can, however, try to be kind to each other and to accept kindness from others.

Rabbinic stories that feature suffering and trauma offer food for thought to us today. There may be times when we can reflect on our experience to uncover and perhaps understand the source of our trauma; at the same time, identifying the source of trauma cannot necessarily erase its impact on our lives. For some, pain and trauma may impel future endeavors, while for others, it may be something we long to have lifted by a caring friend or teacher. At the very least, these stories remind us that trauma is real and needs to be acknowledged and addressed, both personally and communally.

NOTES
1. All translations of Rabbinic texts are by the author.
2. This sentence is found in the Vilna edition of the Talmud, but is missing in some manuscripts.
3. The story appears in a slightly different version in Babylonian Talmud, *Sanhedrin* 108b–109a.
4. *Dikdukei Sof'rim* provides a list of manuscripts that do not have this sentence, as well as compilations that cite the story omitting the sentence.

3

Can Religion Bring Comfort?

The Case for Liturgy

RABBI LAWRENCE A. HOFFMAN, PhD

IT'S A CLUB with more members than any other organization on the planet. There are no dues, but the up-front cost is exorbitant: To qualify for inclusion, you must have part of your life torn away against your will.

The club has many chapters, depending on the nature of the tear. Usually, it is the death of a loved one: a life's partner, in particular, but sometimes a parent, sibling, or child. Sometimes club membership comes from the permanent alienation or departure of a would-be lover. Another chapter is for debilitating chronic illness, a permanent malady that requires constant care and that, even with such care, renders life anywhere from difficult to impossible.

You can belong to more than one chapter. I do. My daughter was diagnosed with intractable epilepsy when she was a teenager; her many brain surgeries left her (as they say, euphemistically) compromised for life. And I lost my wife to cancer just short of three years ago.

Religion is supposed to comfort club members, but does it? C. S. Lewis married late in life, then watched his wife die four years later; even he, an ardent Christian if ever there was one, confessed, "Talk to me about the truth of religion and I'll listen gladly. Talk to me about the duty of religion and I'll listen submissively. But don't come talking to me about the consolations of religion or I will suspect that you don't understand."[1]

People expect religion to answer the question "Why did it happen to me?" Classical Jewish texts do answer that question, but not in a helpful way, because Rabbinic tradition, overall, views suffering as divine chastisement for sin. The earliest Rabbis who added Job to the canon[2] might not have agreed. And one of my favorite Talmudic passages (Babylonian Talmud, *K'tubot* 8b) denies it explicitly. When Rav Chiya bar Abba's son dies, Reish Lakish visits him and charges his interpreter (his *m'turg'man*) to offer comfort. When the interpreter justifies the son's death as a consequence of his father's sins, the Talmud objects: "You came to comfort but you added to the pain!"

Unfortunately, the last word in the debate restates the painful solution: Perhaps the father is eminent enough that he (through the death of his son) has been singled out to atone for the sins of others. Similar responses abound. Through tears of grief, a Roman Catholic woman mourning her husband told me, "God takes the best of every generation to make room on earth for others to take their place." I prefer the Talmud's objection.

No Why, No Meaning, No Faith, No Divine Dice

C. S. Lewis, the Talmudic interpreter, and my Roman Catholic informant are all cases where religious doctrine does not help. But doctrine tends toward necessary truth: Too bad if you don't like it. Truth evokes passion, not compassion. What about prayer? Does liturgy deliver what doctrine cannot? It depends.

The liturgy sometimes answers the "why" question. The Yom Kippur marathon comes quickest to mind: We are sinners (*ashamnu, bagadnu, gazalnu*), and we have no good works to our credit (*ein banu maasim*). The beginning of liturgical comfort is to dispense with such explanations. For suffering, pain, and death, there is neither moral nor theological "why."

There's also no meaning of any sort. Writer Annie Dillard pictures schizophrenics extracting existential meaning from random patterns of puddles after a storm. Psychiatrists take notes on the meanings the schizophrenics extract, from which they diagnose their illness. The psychiatrists' meanings are valid and the schizophrenics' are not—not in the way they imagine, anyway. Unless you are a scientist studying microorganic life in stagnant water, a puddle is just a puddle.[3] Disease and death are simply that: disease and death. There is no higher meaning to them.

It is also absurd to suggest that we get over our pain by developing faith. C. S. Lewis certainly had faith, and when my daughter with epilepsy faced one of her several brain surgeries (none of which ended her seizures), so did I. The night before the operation, I visited the patient next door, a teenage boy with epilepsy, who was unable to do anything except watch childish cartoons and endlessly drop a nerf basketball through a hoop affixed to the end of his bed. "How's your faith?" the boy's mother asked. "You gotta have faith," she insisted, as she looked at her multiply damaged son. "He will someday sit at the right hand of God, and if he is good enough for God, he is good enough for me." She had found her faith in the Bible and in her prayer life, and I say, "Good for her." Such faith is a blessing bestowed, but not something we can necessarily come up with on our own.

As I say, the night before my daughter's operation, I still had faith that God might cure her. But after my conversation with the mother next door, I couldn't help but wonder, "What if God heals my daughter, but not her much worse off son?" Albert Einstein is said to have insisted "God does not play dice with the universe." I concluded that night, "God does not play dice with people's lives." Since God does not answer prayers of healing for everyone, God does not answer prayers of healing for anyone.

Yet I found myself praying anyhow. And I am not alone. True, there are famous exceptions: folk like Bertrand Russell, Sigmund Freud, and more recently the "new atheists" like philosopher Daniel Dennett, who goes so far as to say, "I have had to forgive my friends who were praying for me [when I was sick]. I have resisted the temptation to respond, 'Thanks, I appreciate it, but did you also sacrifice a goat?'"[4] There are multitudes of others, however, who—like me—do not believe that God answers prayer, but who nonetheless join heartily in prayers for healing. Could it be that among the Rabbis of earlier times, there were people like that? Is it likely that we moderns are the first generations to pray for divine healing even though we don't believe in its efficacy? If we are not the first, then perhaps a closer look at our prayers will reveal a theology of prayer that is more nuanced than we normally think.

A Nuanced View of Prayer

I get such a nuanced view from our meal liturgy, especially *Birkat Ha-Mazon* (Blessing After Meals) and its citation of Psalm 37:25, colloquially referred to by its first two Hebrew words, *Naar hayiti*: "I have been young, and now I am old, but I have never seen the righteous abandoned and their children begging for food."[5] Is there any possibility whatsoever that any rabbi anywhere actually believed this?[6] Following the Babylonian Talmud (*Y'vamot* 16b), Rashi and the *Tosafot* cannot figure out who in their right mind would even have said it. They conclude that it must have been authored by some unknown angel. Samuel Edels (also known as Maharsha, a renowned rabbi and Talmudist, 1555–1631), is so astonished by it that he calls it *vadai chidush* (exceptionally novel).[7] It's one thing to read these lines as part of the Biblical canon, where we can agree, disagree, stop to interpret, or even ignore any given verse. But when they are used in liturgy, it doesn't work that way. Take the parallel case of Isaiah 45:7, which praises God, "who makes peace and fashions *evil*," easily explained as Deutero-Isaiah's polemic against Zoroastrian dualism.[8] But when it gets transferred into the liturgy, it is cleaned up to say instead, "who makes peace and fashions *everything*." Liturgy requires assent, not debate.

The *Birkat HaMazon* problem goes beyond *Naar hayiti*. Take the opening blessing, which praises God for "providing food for all." Really? Everyday experience refutes that. One prevalent solution is to translate the Hebrew as a philosophical hypothetical: God does not actually feed everyone, but God is, by definition, the sole Being who could do so. The same solution is offered for other hard-to-believe passages, like "God, who resurrects the dead," which would mean that if there is resurrection, only God has the capacity to do it.

I find that solution disingenuous. Nobody wants to pray that *if* something impossible were to happen, God *would* be the One to do it. And in any event, resurrection is neither confirmable nor deniable, while feeding everyone and never letting children go hungry are matters of empirical observation: It is just not true. Believing that the Sages of old knew that as well as I do, I find it more likely to say that they fashioned prayer not simply as statements of fact (the indicative mood) but as expressions of hope (the optative mood).

Sometimes optative liturgy is framed as petition. At a moment of deep sadness in my own life, I attended an evening service where I was moved to tears while singing *Hashkiveinu*'s opening words, "Lie us down in peace, and raise us up to life." I remember thinking, "Yes, that is indeed what I desire: a peaceful sleep tonight and life renewed tomorrow." At other times, it appears as a statement of fact, as in a hymn I sang with some Christian colleagues at a conference where, again, my life seemed to be falling apart. We offered God various petitions and followed each one with "All will be well, all will be well; all manner of things will be well."⁹ I thought as we sang, "Yes, maybe, somehow, they will be."

Here is where artistry applies. It helps if the medium is music. We will happily sing all sorts of things that would give us pause were we to speak them. If not music, then poetry works well too, because poetry is not empirically deniable. Renaissance poet Sir Philip Sidney put it admirably: "The poet nothing affirmeth and therefore never lieth."¹⁰ Liturgy is akin to Ludwig van Beethoven's Ninth Symphony, Claude Monet's *Water Lilies*, or Robert Frost's "The Road Not Taken." Liturgy is not informational, it is inspirational. It does not tell; it shows. William Shakespeare's Hamlet protests, "There are more things in heaven and on earth, Horatio, than are dreamt of in your philosophy." Liturgy is Hamlet, not Horatio.

What I have said about prayer as optative easily applies to matters like disease, depression, and despair—afflictions of a life still in process, a life where hope is hard to find, but where optative prayer can move us to find it anyway. But we need another approach for the irretrievable loss of a loved one, a condition that never goes away. To be sure, singing our way through *Hashkiveinu* or "All manner of things will be well" can provide some comfort, some hope that our lives will somehow continue despite the felt certainty that they cannot. Perhaps, as well, we may dare to hope to be reunited with our departed loved ones after we too die. But that hope falls short, because when death strikes home, the reunification we want is not in the hereafter but in the here and now, and that is precisely what we cannot have. How, then, does liturgy help mourners face the threat of lifelong loneliness born of deep and irreparable loss?

Here, another characteristic of liturgy matters most—liturgy as expression. Mourners who feel bereft of hope can at least give voice to their anguish. Yet every mourner knows the problem with that. Words fail us—what are we supposed to say? And do people even want to hear it? Liturgy provides a safe and scripted way of sharing how we feel.

Mourners who may feel uncomfortable or unable to inject conversations with their own words of grief are given a liturgical setting in which to do so and a script for that setting, where liturgy, as poetry, expresses the otherwise inexpressible.

Our liturgy has more than its share of poetic reflections on suffering, starting with the psalms. But psalms can be hurtful rather than helpful, because they too are likely to explain suffering as punishment for sin. Instead of asking God to be present in our pain, they try to ameliorate that pain through the possibility of atonement. We should have none of that. Suggesting that people in pain read entire psalms (without our first editing them to omit the verses that stress guilt and atonement) amounts to our rerunning the role of the Talmudic interpreter—coming to comfort but adding to the pain.

Instead of whole psalms, however, individual verses from here and there (technically, a "florilegium") can be strung together. There is plenty of precedent for that strategy. Our early morning *P'sukei D'Zimrah* (*Verses* [!] of Song) must have begun that way: The Cairo Genizah still has instances of that practice, as does the siddur itself (the *K'dushah D'Sidra* [*Uva L'Tziyon Go-eil*], for example).[11] Imagine readings like the following, which organizes individual verses of psalms into a prayer format:

> Out of the depths, I call upon You, O God.
> Why do You stand aloof, uncaring in my time of trouble?
> I am bent and bowed,
> All day long, I stumble about in gloom.
> Every night I drench my bed in tears.
> I am benumbed and crushed,
> Aroar with mental turmoil,
> Weary from groaning.[12]

And beyond the psalms, there is rabbinic liturgy itself. It too is overly obsessed with the nexus between sin and suffering, but in my own life's moment of distress, I drew selectively from the siddur by combining, for example, a line from *Tachanun* and a verse from *Adon Olam*. I used the Hebrew, but English works just as well if it is duly liturgized with poetic license:

> What more can I do, except search You out,
> Hoping for Your kindness?
> In Your hand, I put my soul,
> Whether awake or asleep.
> And with my soul, my body too.
> If You, O God, are with me
> I need not fear.[13]

What we lack is not adequate material, but adequate will to use it creatively. If medieval Judaism was overly fixated on suffering and sin, we modern Jews—especially in the Reform Movement—are obsessed with happiness and health. We advise people in pain to attend services, find community, and feel better. But Shabbat worship is the last place for that to happen. Despite our momentary healing moment, the rest of the service instructs us to be happy. How many services I have attended, in my times of tribulation, where individuals are prompted to share aloud their moments of celebration, of happiness, of gratitude—while I, in my distress, felt only the lack of all three.

I understand the mitzvah of *Oneg Shabbat*. I have no quarrel with it, but we Reform Jews pursue Shabbat joy with too little regard for people in pain. Christian tradition, by contrast, even has a separate category of "Psalms of Lament." Some Christian websites contain instructions on how to write one's own psalm to express mourning, pain, or the helplessness of being unable to relieve the pain of others whom we love the most.

Americans want a religion that is joyous. Ours is. I like it that way. But the genius of religion is its ability to reflect the totality of the human condition, and as much as that condition may be celebratory overall, it is inevitably punctuated with pain as well. From time to time, members of "the club" are relegated to those punctuation marks. We have yet to admit the ubiquity of that suffering and to put a wholehearted effort into developing liturgy for it.

NOTES

1. C. S. Lewis, *A Grief Observed* (HarperOne, 2015), chap. 2, ebook. First published in 1961 by Faber & Faber under the pseudonym N. W. Clerk.
2. For more details on the canonization of the Hebrew Bible, see Lawrence Schiffman, "The Canonization of the Hebrew Scriptures," in *From Text to*

    Tradition: A History of Second Temple and Rabbinic Judaism (Ktav, 1991), 56; reprinted by permission at https://www.myjewishlearning.com/article/creating-the-canon/; and Joel Hoffman, PhD, *On the Bible's Cutting Room Floor: The Holy Scriptures Missing from Your Bible* (Thomas Dunne Books, 2014).

3. Annie Dillard, *Living by Fiction* (Harper Perennial, 2000), 138–39.

4   Daniel Dennett, *I've Been Thinking* (W. W. Norton, 2023), xvi.

5. Translated by the author, loosely based on the translation from *The JPS Tanakh: The Holy Scriptures* (Jewish Publication Society, 1985).

6. Should the children of the righteous get fed, while the children of scoundrels starve? Those rabbis who saw suffering as punishment for sin might have had no problem with it, but it is not morally tenable.

7. See Babylonian Talmud *Y'vamot* 16b; Rashi to Psalm 37:25; *Tosafot* to Babylonian Talmud, *Y'vamot* 16b, d.h. *Pasuk zeh sar haolam amaro*; Maharsha, *Chidushei Aggadot* to Babylonian Talmud, *Y'vamot* 16b, d.h. *ileima kudsha b"h*.

8. Zoroastrianism is an ancient Persian faith still practiced today. Today it claims to be monotheistic, but in antiquity it taught a doctrine of theological dualism, one god of light and good (Ahura Mazda) and another of darkness and evil (Angra Mainyu). When Persia (present-day Iran) conquered Babylonia (present-day Iraq) in 539 BCE, Jews who had been exiled to Babylonia (597–587 BCE) were exposed to Zoroastrian teachings. Deutero-Isaiah is a section of the prophetic Book of Isaiah (chapters 40–55) that scholars believe has a later origin than the rest of Isaiah. Its author, whom we call Deutero-Isaiah (= Second Isaiah) because we do not know his actual name, lived and taught in Zoroastrian Babylonia. He polemicized against Zoroastrian dualism by emphasizing a single God, who, of necessity, must have created all the world as it is—good and bad, light and darkness.

9. Words attributed to fourteenth-century mystic Julian of Norwich, echoing Isaiah 3:10.

10. Gavin Alexander, ed., *Sidney's "The Defence of Poesy" and Selected Renaissance Literary Criticism* (Penguin Books, 2004), 34.

11. The Cairo Genizah is a cache of documents discovered in Cairo that date from the late 800s CE, onward. Jewish prayer books as we know them were largely the product of Jewish authorities in Babylonia (modern-day Iraq) from the ninth and tenth centuries CE. Among the Genizah documents are alternative liturgical customs from the Land of Israel that never made it into that Babylonian-based official order of prayer. The *K'dushah D'Sidra* is a prayer that originated in the Land of Israel but nonetheless did make it into the traditional siddur. It is composed mostly of

a string of Biblical verses. It is also referred to as *Uva L'Tziyon Go-eil*, its opening Hebrew words, which mean "A redeemer will come to Zion."

12. From Psalms 6:7, 10:1, 38:7, 38:9, 130:1. Translated by the author, loosely based on the translations from *The JPS Tanakh*.

13. Translated by the author.

4

Again the Song Goes Out

October 7 Through the Lens of Classic Israeli Song

RABBI WENDY ZIERLER, PhD

> Occasionally, especially when the nation is at war or undergoing some major catastrophe, our poets will speak as a community of voices, each adding his or her voice to a chorus of common concern for human suffering and a common longing for peace on earth. Each speaks in a highly individualistic way, yet contributes his or her unique gift to a larger purpose.
>
> —*Donald Capps*[1]

IN MARCH of 2019 my beloved father, David Zierler, *z"l*, was hit by a truck and killed as he was making his way into a coffee shop to meet a friend. Ten months later, my mother, Marion Zierler, *z"l*, died too. I had been saying *Kaddish* for a full year, first for my dad, then for my mom, when the novel coronavirus engulfed New York and the world, subsuming my personal grief in a larger, worldwide drama. My two consecutive years of *Kaddish* recitation thus became a daily record of the before, during, and after, as it were, of COVID-19 and all of the attendant traumas of 2020.

My academic career has been dedicated to teaching Modern Hebrew and Jewish literature to future rabbis, cantors, and educators, and so much of my work has entailed advocating for the relevance of Modern Hebrew literary texts to Jewish life, learning, and prayer. In the wake of my own experience of personal trauma and grief, I found myself turning to this spiritual conviction about Hebrew poetry as a repository of Torah, theology, and alternative liturgy in a new, urgent, deeply necessary way, as if my religious life depended on it. Early on in my *Kaddish* journey, I adopted a spiritual and pedagogical discipline, each week translating a different prayer-related Hebrew poem and offering commentary in the form of a weekly *d'var Torah*. I dubbed this practice *Shir Chadash shel Yom* (new poem/song of the day), and it has persisted for more than five years now, serving not only as a record of my *Kaddish* and COVID journey—which I have documented in my book *Going Out with Knots: My Two Kaddish Years with Hebrew Poetry* (forthcoming, JPS)—but also of the fear and insecurity of other world events; more recently, it has been focused on the trauma and grief unleashed by the events of October 7, 2023.

Bringing the Hebrew poems and songs of the past to my prayer community in the aftermath of October 7, especially, has been a way for me and my community to recognize our own sorrows, fears, and hopes in those of our Hebrew poetic forebears. The endeavor of translation—of bridging cultural, linguistic, generic, and contextual divides—has served as metaphor for and embodiment of the challenges and opportunities attending the practice of prayer, itself an effort to traverse, however tentatively or incompletely, the impossible distance between ourselves and God. The texts of the poems and songs, themselves, have forged unbearable but also consoling continuities between past and present, between records of earlier traumas and those being experienced now. So many of us believed or hoped that we were moving toward better times, and yet we find ourselves thrown back into many of the same traumas and modes of response from so many decades ago, our current experience now translated and transmitted into the language of the past.

October 7, 2023, fifty years and a day after the Yom Kippur War, completely collapsed the distance between then and now. And so it was that one of the first poems/songs that I taught after that terrible day was a Yom Kippur War song: Naomi Shemer's "B'chol Shanah BaStav, Giora" (Every year in fall, Giora):[2]

Every year in fall, Giora,	בְּכָל שָׁנָה בַּסְּתָו גְּיוֹרָא
The crazy wind in my garden	הָרוּחַ הַמְּטֹרֶפֶת בְּגַנִּי
Cuts down my best roses.	עוֹרֶפֶת אֶת מֵיטַב הַשּׁוֹשַׁנִּים
Every year.	בְּכָל שָׁנָה
Every year in fall, Giora,	בְּכָל שָׁנָה בַּסְּתָו גְּיוֹרָא
I lift my eyes to the mountains	אֶשָּׂא עֵינַי אֶל הֶהָרִים
To see where my help will come	מֵאַיִן יָבוֹא עֶזְרִי
Every year.	בְּכָל שָׁנָה

Every year in fall בְּכָל שָׁנָה בַּסְּתָו
Every year in fall בְּכָל שָׁנָה בַּסְּתָו

You aren't alone, Giora. אַתָּה אֵינְךָ לְבַד גִּיוֹרָא
For in the place where you dwell כִּי בַּמָּקוֹם שֶׁבּוֹ אַתָּה שׁוֹכֵן
Grace and compassion dwell as well. שׁוֹכְנִים הַחֶסֶד וְהַחֵן
And Yechiam still whoops and sings, וְשָׁם יְחִיעָם עוֹד שָׁר לוֹ וּמֵרִיעַ
Tuvia still grows rare black irises, טוּבְיָה מְגַדֵּל עֲדַיִן אִירִיסִים שְׁחוֹרִים וּנְדִירִים
And there you are וְשָׁם אַתָּה
And there are lots of other youngsters וְשָׁם הֲמוֹן הַצְּעִירִים
About whom I said, אֲשֶׁר אָמַרְתִּי
    "My help will come from them." כִּי מֵהֶם יָבוֹא עֶזְרִי

Every year in fall בְּכָל שָׁנָה בַּסְּתָו
Every year in fall בְּכָל שָׁנָה בַּסְּתָו

Every year in fall, Giora, בְּכָל שָׁנָה בַּסְּתָו גִּיוֹרָא
I ask myself אֲנִי שׁוֹאֶלֶת אֶת נַפְשִׁי
When shall I come to dwell there with you? מָתַי אִתְּכֶם לִשְׁכֹּן אָבוֹא
My heart finally resting from its pain. וְנָח לִבִּי מִמַּכְאוֹבוֹ
But every year, Giora, אֲבָל בְּכָל שָׁנָה גִּיוֹרָא
The crazy wind in my garden הָרוּחַ הַמְטֹרֶפֶת בְּגַנִּי
Cuts down my best roses עוֹרֶפֶת אֶת מֵיטַב הַשּׁוֹשַׁנִּים

Every year in fall בְּכָל שָׁנָה בַּסְּתָו
Every year in fall בְּכָל שָׁנָה בַּסְּתָו

Shemer wrote this song in response to the death of Giora Shoham, the son of her close childhood friends, Rut and Shlomo. Giora was twenty-one years old when he was killed after crossing the Suez Canal on October 20, 1973. The song conveys a sense of fatalistic repetition, underscored by the repeated reference to a deranged wind that cuts off the heads of the roses in the speaker's garden. The word *shoshanah* (rose or lily), evokes the allegorical representation of Israel as a *shoshanah bein hachochim*, "a rose among the thorns" (Song of Songs 2:2), and points to the abiding, thorny dangers of life in Israel, while the verb *orefet* (cuts down) calls to mind the Biblical atonement ritual of the *eglah arufah* (the decapitated calf of Deuteronomy 21:1–9), performed in the event that a body of a slain person whose killer is unknown is found in a field. In alluding to this ritual, Shemer hints at the way in which deaths on a battlefield are analogous to those killed "anonymously," leaving communities in need of some ritual of atonement for their inability to bring the killer to justice. The theme of atonement gestures back to the fact of the war having broken out on the Day of Atonement. More specifically, the allusion to the *eglah arufah* acknowledges that there was blame to be placed for the war, and yet it was unclear where to put it; in other words, it acknowledges that the communal leadership needed to do some stocktaking. After the Yom Kippur War, there was widespread sense that *ziknei ha-ir* (the elders of the city) of modern Israel, through lack of readiness and planning and intelligence failures, could not so readily claim, "Our hands have not shed this blood!" How similar those sentiments once again felt in the aftermath of the terrible events of October 7, 2023! How could it be that fifty years later, we were witnessing a surprise attack even more gruesome and calamitous, the result of an even more glaring set of policy and intelligence errors?

So much of the consolation offered in this song is undercut by a sense of unremitting loss. Recalling Psalm 121, one of the series of psalms traditionally recited in cases of illness or times of communal danger, which my community has repeatedly recited as part of thrice-daily prayer since October 7, the speaker in Shemer's song lifts her "eyes to the mountains / To see where my help will come," directly quoting from the first verse of the psalm. She offers comfort to the fallen Giora by saying that he has been laid to rest next to several other promising young men—the kind of men from whom, she had assumed, her own (secular, worldly) help would come, a statement that effectively undermines any hope in future help, divine or otherwise. The speaker again grasps for consolation by declaring that in the place (*bamakom*) where Giora rests *chein vachesed* (grace and compassion) also dwell, the word *bamakom* denoting both a specific burial place as well as *HaMakom*, the name for God used in the traditional formula of consolation offered to a mourner ("May *HaMakom* bring comfort to you among all the mourners of Zion"). Shemer's insistence that Giora has been laid to rest alongside grace and compassion suggests, on the one hand, the abiding presence of these divine attributes, and on the other, the awareness that war tends to eradicate and put to eternal rest any notion of *rachamim* (compassion). Isn't that, too, one of the great sorrows of this time: that fifty years later we've come no closer to ending the cycle of violence, that the deranged winds are now blowing even more strongly than ever before?

One of the other poems/songs that I taught soon after October 7 was Natan Alterman's "Shir HaEmek" (Song of the valley, 1934–35),[3] which captured so perfectly the sudden shift on October 7 from the joy and calm of Simchat Torah to communal tragedy:

Rest comes to the weary	בָּאָה מְנוּחָה לַיָּגֵעַ
And calm to the laborer.	וּמַרְגּוֹעַ לֶעָמֵל.
Pale night spreads out	לַיְלָה חִוֵּר מִשְׂתָּרֵעַ
Upon the fields of the Jezreel Valley.	עַל שְׂדוֹת עֵמֶק יִזְרְעֶאל.
Dew below and moonlight above,[4]	טַל מִלְמַטָּה וּלְבָנָה מֵעַל,
From the Beit Alpha to Nahalal.	מִבֵּית אַלְפָא עַד נַהֲלָל.
Oh, what a night of nights.[5]	מַה, מַה לַיְלָה מִלֵּיל?
Quiet in Jezreel.	דְּמָמָה בְּיִזְרְעֶאל.
Sleep dear valley, glorious land,	נוּמָה עֵמֶק, אֶרֶץ תִּפְאֶרֶת,
We shall stand on guard.[6]	אָנוּ לְךָ מִשְׁמֶרֶת.
The sea of grain is swaying,	יָם הַדָּגָן מִתְנוֹעֵעַ,
The song of the flocks rings out,	שִׁיר הָעֵדֶר מְצַלְצֵל,
This is my country and her fields,	זוֹהִי אַרְצִי וּשְׂדוֹתֶיהָ,
This is the Jezreel Valley.	זֶהוּ עֵמֶק יִזְרְעֶאל.
Be blessed, my land and praised	תְּבֹרַךְ אַרְצִי וְתִתְהַלַּל
From Beit Alpha to Nahalal.	מִבֵּית אַלְפָא עַד נַהֲלָל.
Oh, what a night of nights . . .	מַה, מַה לַיְלָה מִלֵּיל? . . .
Darkness on Mount Gilboa,	אֹפֶל בְּהַר הַגִּלְבּוֹעַ,
A horse gallops from shade to shade.	סוּס דּוֹהֵר מִצֵּל אֶל צֵל.
A holler flies up high.	קוֹל זְעָקָה עָף גָּבוֹהַּ,
Over the fields of the Jezreel Valley.	מִשְּׂדוֹת עֵמֶק יִזְרְעֶאל.
Who just shot? Who just fell?	מִי יָרָה וּמִי זֶה שָׁם נָפַל
Between Beit Alpha and Nahalal.	בֵּין בֵּית אַלְפָא וְנַהֲלָל?
Oh, what a night of nights . . .	מַה, מַה לַיְלָה מִלֵּיל? . . .

"Shir HaEmek" was written for a 1935 Zionist fundraising film sponsored by the Keren Hayesod (Jewish National Fund) entitled *L'Chayim Chadashim* (To new life). It was the third film made in the Land of Israel, and the first with a soundtrack.[7] In the film, composer Daniel Samburskey appears in a kibbutz dining hall and teaches the song to the members of the kibbutz, after which we see various *kibbutznikim* singing the song as they do their respective jobs—an illustration of a new kind of collective workers' life on the land. Two agricultural settlements are mentioned in the song: Beit Alfa, the first Shomer HaTza-ir kibbutz, which sits on the site of an ancient synagogue, and Nahalal, the first worker's settlement in the Jezreel Valley. Together they are meant to exemplify the Zionist movement and its ancient historical basis.

The poem—a lullaby to the land and a paean to the collectivist ethos of the kibbutz—describes the pastoral calm at nighttime in that ancient historical Jezreel Valley, a sense of serenity underscored by the allusions to the manna in the desert and the double portion given to the people on Shabbat. Exodus 16:32 commands that one portion of this manna be forever safeguarded (a *mishmeret*) as a reminder of how God provided for the people of Israel in the desert. Alterman's use here of the word *mishmeret* repurposes this language of God's providing for the people in the desert as a way of declaring the Zionist activist commitment to standing on guard and protecting the land. Indeed, one way to read the poem is as a description of the valley from the point of view of one of its *shom'rim* (guards).

The film, produced for Zionist publicity and fundraising purposes, did not include what appears here as the third stanza, which describes a sudden shooting in the dark. This tragic turn is characteristic of much of Alterman's poetry, a type of writing that is steeped in the awareness of the Jewish experiences of sudden persecution, war, and death.

I used to laugh at this seemingly discordant stanza. What was it doing there in the midst of such a gorgeous, bucolic song? Can we not sing something beautiful that is untainted with evil and fear? That was before October 7. These days, I'm no longer laughing; this stanza perfectly expresses the shock we all felt that day. Right in the midst of our joyous celebration of the holidays of Sh'mini Atzeret and Simchat Torah came this horrendous attack against the southern kibbutzim, several of whose members were social justice and peace activists. The State of Israel is supposed to be a place of refuge for the Jews, but even there, as Alterman's poetry attests, danger can strike at any time, the Zionist project hinging on an ongoing willingness to give one's life in defense of the nation. This sense of danger or potential war is also implicit in the setting of the poem in the gorgeous, historic Jezreel Valley, site of the battles of Deborah and Barak and of the tragic deaths of King Saul and his sons.

And in the same way that the outcome of the attack in the poem remains ambiguous and unclear—who fired and who fell, one of ours or theirs?—we remained unclear in those early days about what awaited Israel and the world in the aftermath of October 7, a date that like 9/11 would now live on in historical infamy. What awaited the hundreds of thousands of Israeli soldiers who'd been mobilized and were now standing on *mishmeret* (guard) in the south or in the north? What was it going to take to restore the nighttime vista of calm, of swaying grains, and of holiday peace to Israel, to Diaspora Jewry, and to the world?

Then came the ground invasion, and shortly thereafter the rally in Washington to return the hostages. All of this thrust us back into modes and experiences that we had previously identified with the distant past. Once again, Israel was fighting a war after a surprise attack on a holy day. Once again, worldwide Jewry was dealing with alarming levels of antisemitism and anti-Jewish violence. And once again, like decades ago, during the time of the struggle for Soviet Jewry, we found ourselves gathering en masse in Washington to let out a cry of protest, conscience, and solidarity for those imprisoned in a foreign land. Veritable convoys of car drivers, bus riders, and airplane travelers had made their way from cities and communities all across the country to join the march. And when we got there, one of the things we did was sing with Yishai Ribo, Omer Adam, even Matisyahu. Once again, as in Zionist days of yore, we are compiling a war soundtrack: old and new songs together serving as the conduits and carriers of our collective pains and hopes.

It was after the Washington rally that I presented Natan Yonatan's "Shayarah Shelanu" (Our convoy, lyrics 1948, music 1957–58), a poem that hinges on the idea of returning to old modes and on the association of military convoys with caravans of poetry and song:[8]

Again the song goes out on its way	שׁוּב יוֹצֵא הַזֶּמֶר אֶל הַדֶּרֶךְ
Again our days keep on weeping	שׁוּב הוֹלְכִים יָמֵינוּ וּבוֹכִים
Convoy, where are you passing?	שַׁיָּרָה, אֶל אָנָה אַתְּ עוֹבֶרֶת?
Convoy, sad upon the paths.	שַׁיָּרָה, עָצוּב עַל הַדְּרָכִים.

Again you're carrying country bread and water	שׁוּב נוֹשֵׂאת אַתְּ פַּת-קֶבֶר וּמַיִם
Satchels, sorrow of expanses.	תַּרְמִילִים, תּוּגָה שֶׁל מֶרְחָבִים.
Again you hang eyes on the heavens	שׁוּב תּוֹלָה אַתְּ עַיִן בַּשָּׁמַיִם
And a path upon the starry lane.	וּמִשְׁעוֹל בִּנְתִיב הַכּוֹכָבִים.
Darkness; only singing sound of weapons	עֲלָטָה; רַק קוֹל רִנַּת-הַנֶּשֶׁק
Somewhere on the sealed path.	אֵי בְּזֶה הַדֶּרֶךְ חֲסוּמָה.
You, my convoy, of unveiled eyes[9]	אַתְּ, שַׁיָּרָתִי, גְּלוּיַת-עֵינַיִם
Only the mortal bullet is blind!	רַק כַּדּוּר-הַמָּוֶת הוּא סוּמָא!

"Shayarah Shelanu" was written in 1948 by a twenty-five-year-old Natan Klein (later known as Natan Yonatan), in memory of Aharon Agassi, an immigrant from Iraq and a Shomer HaTza-ir kibbutz member, who was killed near the present-day Israeli moshav of Shoresh on January 9, 1948, while bringing agricultural supplies to Jerusalem. The song commemorates the heroic effort to send truck convoys to supply bread, water, and other necessities to Jerusalem during that time of war and siege. The third and final stanza of the poem/song (in this particular iteration) tells the tragic ending to the story: The road is blocked (*chasumah*) by the enemy; Agassi is trapped. The convoy's errand is righteous and prophetic; indeed, it is described by the speaker as *g'luyat einayim* (of unveiled eyes)—an expression borrowed from the beginning of Balaam's prophecy in Numbers 24:4, denoting clear-eyed prophetic vision. And yet, the enemy bullets prove to be both morally and lethally blind (*suma*, a tragic rhyme with *chasumah*, sealed), and the hero, Aharon, is killed.

As part of this elegiac storytelling, Natan Yonatan plays on the dual meanings of the root *zayin-mem-reish*, meaning both "to sing" and "to prune or cut down," and of the word *shayarah*, meaning both "convoy" and "enduring remnant"; there is also the visual similarity between the words *shayarah* (convoy) and *shirah* (song, a synonym for the word *zemer*). Natan Yonatan personifies both in the feminine, intimately asking her/ them, "Where are you going? To what sad place on the side of the road?" Metaphorically speaking, then, the poem is about convoys of feeling being set into motion as a consequence of war and loss: veritable caravans of grief, one vehicle of sadness following and supplying the other.

There is something so soul crushing about this return to such dark places and modes of loss. It is nothing short of devastating that this 1948 song feels so immediate and relevant in the present moment. And yet, there is something so utterly inspiring about the Israeli and Jewish ability to turn grief into song and solidarity—not for the purpose of wallowing in it, but as a way of envisioning a path for the enduring caravan of Israel to continue its lifesaving, life-affirming mission. In the context of Zionist return to Israel, Modern Hebrew poetry—set to music and sung at kibbutz sing-alongs and other *arvei shirah* (song evenings)—came to substitute for traditional public prayer; Hebrew songs served as a nostalgic "remnant of synagogue culture."[10] It is no accident, I would argue, that "Shayarah Shelanu" became the standard opening song for so many of these *shirah b'tzibur* (public sing-along) events, including the annual song festival at Kibbutz Ein Gev.[11] It is no accident that "Shuv Yotzei HaZemer" (Again the song goes out), as the song has more recently been renamed, serves as the opening song of one of *1000 Zemer V'Od Zemer* (A thousand and one songs),[12] the songbook that my husband Daniel and I use every Shabbat morning when we sing to his mom at her memory care facility, as these classic Hebrew songs are one of the few ways we have to connect with her, given her advanced stage of Alzheimer's. "Shayarah Shelanu/Shuv Yotzei HaZemer" is one of those songs that has the capacity to bring people back—not just to a shared sense of tragedy, but to a feeling of unity and purpose. None of us wants to suffer trauma or loss or to be back in this dark place of war, but we can take some solace in what Donald Capps refers to in the epigraph to this essay as our "chorus of common concern"—in this case, our ability to find ourselves in Hebrew poems and songs of the past, to sing together, cry out in protest together, and affirm together that the Jewish *shayarah* of sustenance and song will keep going on, God willing, until all grief is turned forever into gladness.

NOTES

1. Donald Capps, introduction to *The Poet's Gift: Toward the Renewal of Pastoral Care* (Westminster John Knox Press, 1993), 4.
2. © Naomi Shemer and ACUM. See https://www.youtube.com/watch?v=OS9uUlfBrbA.

3. © Natan Alterman and ACUM. See https://www.youtube.com/watch?v=jPLZTOfhk8w.

4. See *Yalkut Shimoni* 260 on Exodus 16, כְּתִיב וַתַּעַל שִׁכְבַת הַטָּל וּכְתִיב וּבְרֶדֶת הַטָּל טַל מִלְמַעְלָה וְטַל מִלְמַטָּה, "As it is written, 'when the fall of dew lifted' [Exodus 16:14] and 'when the dew fell' [Numbers 11:9]. [This indicates] dew from above and dew from below."

5. See Isaiah 21:11, שֹׁמֵר מַה מִלַּיְלָה שֹׁמֵר מַה מִלֵּיל, "A call comes to me from Seir: 'Watchman, what of the night? Watchman, what of the night?'"

6. See Exodus 16:32, "Moses said, 'This is what the Eternal has commanded: Let one *omer* of it be kept *mishmeret* throughout the ages, in order that they may see the bread that I fed you in the wilderness when I brought you out from the land of Egypt.'"

7. The song is available to hear at https://www.youtube.com/watch?v=CX-7aeyv_ASs from 0:28.

8. © Natan Yonatan and ACUM. The entirety of "Shayara Shelanu" was originally published in *Al HaMishmar* newspaper on May 4, 1948. See https://www.youtube.com/watch?v=aLENoqCeF7U.

9. See Numbers 24:4–5, "Word of one who hears God's speech, / Who beholds visions from the Almighty, / Prostrate, but with **eyes unveiled** (*g'luy einayim*): / How fair are your tents, O Jacob, / Your dwellings, O Israel!"

10. Oz Almog, *The Sabra: The Creation of the New Jew* (University of California Press, 2000), 236. For a discussion of sing-alongs in the context of Israeli emigrants to New York, see Moshe Shokeid, "The People of the Song," in *Children of Circumstances: Israeli Emigrants in New York* (Cornell University Press, 1988), 104–25.

11. See https://www.youtube.com/watch?v=UOoSikY-Lqg.

12. Telma Eligon and Rafi Pesachson, eds., *1000 Zemer V'Od Zemer* (Masada, 1981).

5

Speaking About the Unspeakable

Prayers from the Gaza War

RABBI DALIA MARX, PHD

Translated by Rabbi Ari Vernon

OCTOBER 7, 2023, was the day of the horrific attack by the terror-ist organization Hamas against Israel and its people. This attack claimed about twelve hundred Israeli and foreigner lives—innocent men, women, children, infants, elderly, civilians all—injured many hundreds more, and led to the kidnapping of 251 people to the Gaza Strip. The violence spread from kibbutzim and small towns in the west-ern Negev to a peace festival taking place nearby. It was unprecedented and unimaginable, as was the war that followed. Unfortunately, as I write these words, the war has not yet ended. It may seem that words could not possibly encapsulate the unimaginable catastrophe or give voice to the unspeakable events we have endured. And yet, just as the catastrophe was unprecedented in the history of the State of Israel, so was the liturgical response that followed.

Though the saying attributed to the Roman leader Cicero is that "when cannons thunder, the muses fall silent," the reality is that times of stress, uncertainty, and fear are often characterized by an outburst of creativity, both literary and liturgical. This chapter is thus somewhat of an ad hoc reflection on prayers resulting from the war. Not enough time has passed for a full consideration of the liturgical creativity that has begun and continues in response to the Gaza War. Consider this an initial testimony and experimental investigation of those efforts.

Jews have long grappled with crises and tragedies with liturgy and rit-ual as the touchstone for the challenges of their lives. Numerous Jewish historical experiences rise from within the prayer books, and one can see them as a diary of the life of the people of Israel, as liturgy scholar Jakob Petuchowski described it.[1] This does not mean that every single experience of the nation is encompassed in prayer books, and indeed it is interesting to investigate which events were deemed worthy of yielding liturgical fruit. As a gross generalization, it can be said that more recent events and the liturgy created in response have rarely earned a place in our canon, even if liturgical creativity hasn't stopped. However, even if new prayers haven't achieved canonical status, prayer and *piyut* (liturgical poetry) have been composed throughout the generations as a response to crises and tragedy.

The realm of prayer is where the murmurings of the heart, hopes, and fears find expression. The fixed and obligatory prayers are not in and of themselves connected to life's circumstances, so we can expect to see the influence of significant events on prayer, its language, and its implementation, particularly since prayers are perhaps Judaism's most central locus for our discourse with God, spirit, immediate community, and even *K'lal Yisrael* (the entire Jewish people) in both the present and past. This, combined with the ease and accessibility of distributing texts thanks to digital-age tools, explains the centrality of prayer in this moment as well. If, in the past, rabbinic figures or important communities published formal prayers following significant events—sometimes years after those events had passed—creativity now comes from the public in a variety of ways in the moment itself.

Previous Israeli wars were also characterized by creativity in songs and hymns in the Israeli context, though in no previous war or national crisis has the momentum of ritual and liturgical creativity been as intense as that which has appeared following the Simchat Torah massacre and the war that followed. The language of prayer and *piyut* is the central Jewish language for processing and coping, and it is finding expression not just in traditionally observant communities that are accustomed to fixed and obligatory prayer, but in broader and widening circles in Israel. The shock and helplessness alongside the desire to act led many to express the yearning and pain of their hearts, their sadness and hope, through prayer, poetry, and supplications. I have so far collected over three hundred liturgical texts that were written in the wake of the Simchat Torah massacre and the Gaza War. I have entrusted my collection to the Israeli National Library's project of preserving and gathering information about the Gaza War.

The critical choice to use canonical Jewish language and idiom in political and public contexts demands focused and comprehensive study, as noticeable religious content is being expressed in ever-widening circles. For example, public *Havdalah* services were held by Israeli Reform rabbis and leaders before every Saturday night demonstration in Jerusalem and Tel Aviv during the protest movement against what was referred to as "the judicial revolution" throughout 2023, and they continued during the protest demonstrations during the war. It is possible that the prominence of Jewish liturgical language is the result of the maturation of what has been called *hitchadshut y'hudit* (Jewish revival) in its forms and styles. This may come from a desire to reclaim Jewish language from more conservative and nationalist voices.

This liturgical innovation should be understood as having a collective dimension intended to process and give meaning to events in a broader context. They reflect reality, but they also fashion reality in the consciousness of their creators and consumers. The examples in this chapter are just a small sampling of a larger collection of an impressive range of prayers, *piyutim*, and supplications written after October 7. They differ in character and style, but one can see in them the product of a broad *beit midrash* (house of study), and perhaps they may serve as an initial road map for describing the spiritual-creative responses to the massacre and the war that followed.

Liturgical Creativity Following Crises and Disasters

Texts and rituals written in response to national crises and disasters generally serve three different functions. The first connects to the past. Memory is one of the roles of liturgy, as in the *Avodah* Service, which broadly recalls the service of the High Priest on Yom Kippur. Memory of the past—especially in the context of painful disasters—enables commemoration of victims and gives meaning to their lives as well as their deaths.

The second function of creative liturgy is to help survivors and the broader community cope with the extreme circumstances that have befallen them and their communities. Contextualizing an event through religious ritual can help process these extreme events. In addition, recalling painful events and reviewing them ritually can provide a sense of control over events that render survivors powerless. We see this in many traditional laments that justify God's "harsh decree" as resulting from our own sins; paradoxically, this comforts the survivors because it reinforces the idea that justice and order govern our world.

Finally, liturgy asks for future redemption and expresses a vision for a desired future. For example, many laments and *piyutim* of *S'lichot* conclude with expressions of faith in future redemption, anchored in prophetic language of reward and punishment. They seem to say that there must be a limit to God's punishment, and the request is to merit that we see redemption soon.[2]

Categorizing Liturgical Responses to Tragedy

In her book *Writing Plague: Jewish Responses to the Great Italian Plague*,[3] Susan Einbinder suggests dividing liturgical responses to crisis and tragedy into three categories: new uses of existing texts, processing and interpretation of existing liturgical texts, and creation of new prayers. This is true of the current moment of crisis in Israel.

New Uses of Existing Texts

An example of a new use of existing texts is the supplication known as *v'Acheinu*—"As for our brethren, the entire house of Israel"—traditionally recited during the weekday Torah service. This prayer stands out for earning popularity in many congregations, especially with the melody of American Cantor Abie Rotenberg (sometimes with the addition of *v'achyoteinu*, "and our sisters," to be inclusive).

Interpretation of Existing Texts

The prayer-poem of the Israeli judge Or Adam serves as an example of an interpretation of existing liturgy. Judge Adam is a member of the civic kibbutz in Sderot, a city hit hard by the events of Simchat Torah. He published his poem—a kind of poetic midrash on the Passover Haggadah—just before Passover 2024 and titled it "B'chol Dor VaDor," "In Every Generation," which comes from the Passover Haggadah: "In every generation, one must see themself as if they themself left Egypt." The poem demands that its readers put themselves in the place of those who were affected by the massacre, just like the Haggadah asks us to identify with the travails of the Israelites who left Egypt. In these types of interpretive texts, the authors' foundational assumption is that the public recognizes the texts upon which the new hymns and *piyutim* are based. These interpretive texts sometimes adopt the authority of the canonical text, whether they are based upon it or in polemic against it.

בְּכָל דּוֹר וָדוֹר

הַשּׁוֹפֵט אוֹר אָדָם (שְׂדֵרוֹת)

בְּכָל דּוֹר וָדוֹר, חַיָּב אָדָם לִרְאוֹת אֶת עַצְמוֹ כְּאִלּוּ הוּא יָצָא מִמִּצְרַיִם.
כָּל אֶחָד הָיָה עֶבֶד, מִמִּצְרַיִם יָצָא
וְיַזְכִּיר לָנוּ זֹאת לֶחֶם עֹנִי: מַצָּה
שֶׁנֵּדַע לְשַׁמֵּר, גַּם בְּלִי חֹשֶׁךְ וָדָם
אֶת אוֹתָהּ הַחֵרוּת שֶׁל אָדָם וְאָדָם.

בְּכָל דּוֹר וָדוֹר, חַיָּב אָדָם לִרְאוֹת אֶת עַצְמוֹ כְּאִלּוּ הוּא הָיָה בִּכְפַר עַזָּה
כָּל אֶחָד הִסְתַּגֵּר בִּממ"ד בְּשַׁבָּת
כְּשֶׁבַּחוּץ הַטֶּרוֹר הִשְׁתּוֹלֵל וְחָבַט
כָּל אֶחָד הִתְפַּלֵּל צְעָקָה שֶׁלֹּא גְזֵזָה
בַּקִּבּוּץ הֶחָלָל אֶל מוּל שַׁעַר עַזָּה

בְּכָל דּוֹר וָדוֹר, חַיָּב אָדָם לִרְאוֹת אֶת עַצְמוֹ כְּאִלּוּ הוּא חָלָל בְּרֵעִים
כָּל אֶחָד מֵאִתָּנוּ לֹא הֵבִין מָה זֶה כָּאן
כְּשֶׁהַיְרִי חָדַר אֶת הַלַּמּוֹת מוּסִיקָה
וְלִרְאוֹת אֶת עַצְמוֹ נוֹפֵל מַטָּה מִגְּבֹהַּ
כָּל אֶחָד מֵאִתָּנוּ נֶאֱנַס שָׁם בַּנּוֹבָה

בְּכָל דּוֹר וָדוֹר, חַיָּב אָדָם לִרְאוֹת אֶת עַצְמוֹ כְּאִלּוּ הוּא נֶחְטַף מִנִּיר עַז
הַחֻרְבָּן, הַשְּׂרֵפָה, אֵימִים הַמַּרְאוֹת
כָּל אֶחָד עַל הַטֶּנְדֶר עִם יָדַיִם קְשׁוּרוֹת
וְאֵימָה בַּפָּנִים שֶׁל נָשִׁים וְשֶׁל טַף
בְּכָל דּוֹר וָדוֹר מִנִּיר עַז אַתָּה נֶחְטַף

בְּכָל דּוֹר וָדוֹר, חַיָּב אָדָם לִרְאוֹת אֶת עַצְמוֹ בּוֹנֶה אֶת בְּאֵרִי
כָּל אֶחָד בְּכָל זְמַן עוֹד יָקוּם מֵעָפָר
יִנְשֹׁךְ אֶת שְׂפָתָיו וְיָשׁוּב אֶל הַסְּפָר
יֵצֵא מִמִּצְרַיִם יִתְגַּבֵּר כַּאֲרִי
מֵי-חַיִּים עוֹד יִרְווּ מֵאוֹתָהּ בְּאֵרִי.

בְּכָל דּוֹר וָדוֹר, חַיָּב אָדָם לִרְאוֹת אֶת עַצְמוֹ כְּאִלּוּ הוּא יָצָא מִמִּצְרַיִם

In Every Generation
Judge Or Adam (Sderot)

In every generation, one must see themselves as if they themself left Egypt.
Everyone was a slave, from Egypt they fled
We're reminded of it by affliction—poor bread
We should know to guard, without blood or dark
The same freedom of each human heart.

In every generation, one must see themselves as if they themself were in
  [kibbutz] Kfar Aza.
Everyone in saferooms on Shabbat was shut
As outside terror went wild and struck
All praying in shouts unending
Facing the gates of Gaza from the defiled kibbutz.

In every generation, one must see themself as if they were defiled
  at Re'im.
None of us understood what was here
When the gunfire pierced the musical beat
To see themself from on high fall
We were all raped at the Nova festival.

In every generation, one must see themself as if they were taken hostage
  at Nir Oz.
The destruction, the burning, the threats, the sights
In the back of the truck with their hands tied
Women and children with horror-filled faces
In every generation from Nir Oz you are taken.

In every generation, one must see themself building Be'eri.
Everyone will eventually rise from the dust
Bite their lip and return to the kibbutz on the border
Leave Egypt, Be'eri overcome[4]
Life-giving water that same well will run.

In every generation, one must see themselves as if they themself left Egypt.

New Liturgical Texts

An example of new prayers are the countless prayers for the refugees and captives that were written in many circles in Israeli society. Each is stamped by the ideology and theology of its writer. The first is a *r'shut* (petitionary) prayer by Rabbi Shira Levine, and the other is a prayer for the hostages written by Reform Rabbi Oded Mazor.

רְשׁוּת

הָרַבָּה שִׁירָה לֵוִין

עַל דַּעַת הַמָּקוֹם וְעַל דַּעַת הַקָּהָל

בִּישִׁיבָה שֶׁל מַטָּה וּבִישִׁיבָה שֶׁל מַעְלָה

לִכְבוֹד כָּל אֵלֶּה שֶׁהָלְכוּ לְפָנַי

הֲרֵינִי נִכְנֶסֶת לִתְפִלָּה זֹאת בְּלֵב שָׁבוּר וּבְיִרְאָה.

בְּשָׁעָה שֶׁשַּׁעֲרֵי הַשָּׁמַיִם פְּתוּחִים

נִתְפַּלֵּל בְּתִקְוָה לִישׁוּעָה בִּמְהֵרָה וּבִזְמַן קָרוֹב

נִתְפַּלֵּל לְהַמְתָּקַת הַדִּינִים

נִתְפַּלֵּל לַהֲשָׁבַת הַחֲטוּפִים

שְׁלוֹמֵנוּ קָשׁוּר בְּחוּט לִשְׁלוֹמָם.ן!

אָנָּא ה' עֲשֵׂה לְמַעֲנָם.ן אִם לֹא לְמַעֲנֵנוּ.

יִהְיוּ לְרָצוֹן אִמְרֵי פִינוּ וְהֶגְיוֹן לִבֵּנוּ.

Permission
Rabbi Shira Levine

"With the consent of the Almighty
and consent of this congregation
in a convocation of the heavenly court
and a convocation of the lower court . . ."[5]
In honoring those who passed before me
I hereby enter this service with a broken heart and with awe.
At this time, when the gates of heaven are open,
Let us pray for swift deliverance in near time
Let us pray to sweeten the harsh decree
Let us pray for the return of the hostages
Our well-being is tied to theirs![6]
Please, Eternal, do this for their behalf if not for ours.
May the words of our mouths and the meditation of our hearts
   be acceptable to You.[7]

תְּפִלָּה לִשְׁמִירַת, הַצָּלַת וַהֲשָׁבַת הַחֲטוּפוֹת.ים וְהַשְּׁבוּיִּים.וֹת
הָרַב עוֹדֵד מָזוֹר

מִי שֶׁבֵּרַךְ אֲבוֹתֵינוּ וְאִמּוֹתֵינוּ, אַבְרָהָם וְשָׂרָה, רִבְקָה וְיִצְחָק, רָחֵל, יַעֲקֹב וְלֵאָה,
מִי שֶׁעָנָה לְדִינָה בְּבֵית מְעַנֶּיהָ, לְיוֹסֵף בְּבֵית הָאֲסוּרִים וּלְדָנִיֵּאל בְּגוֹב הָאֲרָיוֹת,
אֱלֹהֵי אָבִינוּ אַבְרָהָם, הָרִאשׁוֹן שֶׁחֵרַף נַפְשׁוֹ לִשְׁחְרוּרָם שֶׁל שְׁבוּיִים וַחֲטוּפִים –
הוּא יְבָרֵךְ אֶת כָּל הַשְּׁבוּיִים וְהַשְּׁבוּיוֹת אֲשֶׁר נֶחְטְפוּ בִּידֵי אוֹיֵב, וְאֶת כָּל
הַנֶּעְדָּרִים וְהַנֶּעֱדָרוֹת, אֶזְרָחִים, חַיָּלִים, בָּנוֹת וּבְנֵי אָדָם, [כָּאן נִתָּן לְהַזְכִּיר שֵׁמוֹת]
הַנְּתוּנִים בְּצָרָה וּבַשִּׁבְיָה.
יְהִי רָצוֹן מִלְּפָנֶיךָ, יְיָ צְבָאוֹת, שֶׁתִּפְדֶּם בִּמְהֵרָה מִשֶּׁבִי וְתַחְזִירֵם לְאַרְצָם,
לְמִשְׁפְּחְתָּם וּלְבֵיתָם, בְּרִיאִים וּשְׁלֵמִים בְּגוּפָם וּבְרוּחָם. הַשְׁכֵּן תַּעֲצוּמוֹת תִּקְוָה
בְּלֵב יַקִּירֵיהֶם הַמְיַחֲלִים לְשׁוּבָם בִּדְאָגָה טְרוּפָה. תֵּן תְּבוּנָה בְּלֵב הָעֲמֵלִים
לְשִׁחְרוּרָם וְרַחֲמִים בְּלֵב שׁוֹבֵיהֶם.
הַמָּקוֹם יְרַחֵם עֲלֵיהֶם, וְיוֹצִיאֵם מִצָּרָה לִרְוָחָה, וּמֵאֲפֵלָה לְאוֹרָה, וּמִשִּׁעְבּוּד
לִגְאֻלָּה, הַשְׁתָּא בַּעֲגָלָא וּבִזְמַן קָרִיב, וִיקֻיַּם בָּהֶם הַכָּתוּב: "קוֹל בְּרָמָה נִשְׁמָע נְהִי
בְּכִי תַמְרוּרִים רָחֵל מְבַכָּה עַל בָּנֶיהָ מֵאֲנָה לְהִנָּחֵם עַל בָּנֶיהָ כִּי אֵינֶנּוּ: כֹּה אָמַר יְיָ,
מִנְעִי קוֹלֵךְ מִבֶּכִי וְעֵינַיִךְ מִדִּמְעָה כִּי יֵשׁ שָׂכָר לִפְעֻלָּתֵךְ נְאֻם יְיָ וְשָׁבוּ מֵאֶרֶץ אוֹיֵב:
וְיֵשׁ תִּקְוָה לְאַחֲרִיתֵךְ נְאֻם יְיָ וְשָׁבוּ בָנִים וּבָנוֹת לִגְבוּלָם" (יִרְמְיָהוּ טו-יז)
וְנֹאמַר אָמֵן.

A Prayer for Guarding, Redeeming, and Freeing the Hostages
Rabbi Oded Mazur
Translation by Rabbi Naamah Kelman

May the One who blessed our ancestors: Abraham and Sarah, Isaac and Rebekah, Jacob, Rachel and Leah,

May the One who answered Dina in her torture, Joseph in prison, and Daniel in the Lion's Den,

God of Abraham, the first, who was willing to risk his life for the release of prisoners and hostages.

May this God bless the hostages, taken captive by our enemy, and all those missing and unaccounted for: citizens, soldiers, men, women, and children [add names] who are imprisoned and in grave danger.

May it be Your will, God of All, that they be released speedily and returned to our land, to their families and to their homes, safe and sound in body and in spirit. Plant the power of hope in the hearts of their loved ones frantic and yearning for their release. Grant wisdom in the hearts of those laboring for their release, and compassion in the hearts of their captors.

May God's presence spread mercy on them and save them from
trouble to well-being, from darkness to light, from enslavement to
redemption.

May it be swift and speedily, as it is written in Jeremiah: "Thus said
God: A cry is heard in Ramah—wailing, bitter weeping—Rachel
weeping for her children. She refuses to be comforted for her children,
who are gone. Thus said God: Restrain your voice from weeping,
your eyes from shedding tears; for there is a reward for your labor—
declares God: They shall return from the enemy's land" (Jeremiah
31:15–17).

And let us say: AMEN.

The creativity in response to the October 7 massacre and the war
that broke out in its aftermath reflects a range of theological, ideological, and literary-stylistic references to bodies of prayer that exist within
Jewish tradition. Some were written in the spirit of extant prayers and
hymns, and others are original compositions. All of them come from
complex positions of faith, defiance, despair, and hope.

"Ephemeral" Prayers

Will prayers and supplications written in response to extreme crises find
a place in prayer books or the ritual service of various synagogues? What
can we foresee for the integration and assimilation of prayers even in
the changing tides of religious practice? If we compare texts that relate
directly to specific events, as opposed to those that use general and
generic language, we'll see that prayers and supplications with specific-
ity tend not to enter into the customary liturgy, and those with more
general language are likely to find themselves in prayer books. *Piyutim*
that graphically describe the harrowing crimes of the Crusaders against
the Jews in the Rhineland in the eleventh through thirteenth centuries,
for example, were not widely included in the regular prayer service,
but another contemporarily written prayer, *Av HaRachamim* (Compassionate One),[8] which calls on God to recall "the holy communities that
gave their lives for the sanctification of the Divine Name" and asks for
"vengeance for the spilled blood of God's servants," was included in
European prayer books and is recited on some Shabbats after the Torah

reading. The general and generic language of this prayer, whose author is unknown, weaves the sacrifice of the murdered into Jewish and general human experience. Perhaps for that reason it was found appropriate to recite on Shabbat in synagogue over many generations.

As with journalism, liturgy can be as ephemeral as the newsflashes updated hourly on a news website. The news may be of great importance and may raise issues through its immediacy and accuracy, but by the next day it has lost its value. Careful critical assessment, usually made after some time, is what gives a text authority and canonical status. When analyzing prayers and songs that were written before, during, and after the process of disengagement from Gush Katif in Gaza in 2005, I drew attention to the fact that texts expressing the harshness of the immediate experience did not generally survive. However, several of the texts that used more general language that could apply to a range of situations (political, historical, spiritual) earned a longer lifespan.

This is only an initial assessment of some of the liturgical responses to the October 7 massacre and the subsequent war in Gaza. This assessment is being made as the war continues, and we hope to soon be able to speak of it in the past tense. This is undoubtedly not the last work on this topic, but I hope that by identifying and sorting these initial attempts there will be some benefit for understanding our current events and perhaps also for understanding the broader phenomenon of liturgical creativity in the face of extreme circumstances. Time will tell what the lifespan of these and similar texts will be.

I pray that new prayers will very soon be needed for happier and better times to come.

NOTES

A more detailed and comprehensive version of this chapter will be published in a Festschrift for Professor Uri Ehrlich (in Hebrew). I thank the translator, Rabbi Ari Vernon, and the editor, Rabbi Anne Villarreal-Belford, for their tremendous help, making this content available for English readers.

1. Jakob J. Petuchowski, *Prayerbook Reform in Europe* (World Union for Progressive Judaism 1968), 22–23.

2. For more details, please see Rabbi Dalia Marx, PhD, "Liturgical Responses to Catastrophe: A Preliminary Outline," *CCAR Journal* (Spring 2022): 75–91.

3. Susan Einbinder, *Writing Plague: Jewish Responses to the Great Italian Plague* (University of Pennsylvania Press, 2022).

4. The wordplay with the name Be'eri, meaning "my well," is difficult to capture in translation. When used with reference to a well or spring, the verb form of this word can also mean "overflow."

5. Citation of the introduction to *Kol Nidrei*, recited on Yom Kippur.

6. Levine alludes to a well-known poem by the poet Zelda, שלומי קשור בחוט אל שלומך ("My well-being is attached with a string to yours").

7. Based on Psalm 19:15.

8. *Av HaRachamim* translates literally as "Compassionate Father." This term combines masculine and feminine imagery by pairing *Av* (Father) with *Rachamim* (compassion), whose Hebrew root (*rechem*) means "womb."

PART TWO

Trauma of Acute and Chronic Illness

6

Every Challenge Is a Journey
What I Learned from Chronic Cancer

Rabbi Lindsey Danziger

I LIVE WITH CHRONIC, incurable cancer. When I touch my body in certain places, I can feel it. When I look in the mirror at certain angles, I can see it. Lurking just below the surface of my skin is the thing that slowly but surely is trying to kill me. I wake up every day, I wash dishes, I drive kids to dance class, I host Zoom meetings, I wear sunscreen, and at some point, I inevitably contemplate my own death. Inside, my B cells gradually divide, replicate, and mutate; outside, life goes on and nobody can tell.

It all began one unremarkable summer evening. My husband, Michael, and I were in the bathroom together bathing our two small children, then one- and two-years-old, before bedtime. I decided to take a quick shower myself. As I washed my body, I noticed a large, soft lump below my hip bone. I got out of the shower, and Michael confirmed a visible swelling. A lifelong hypochondriac, I had been preparing for this moment since childhood! I went to the doctor the next day, who saw that it was a swollen lymph node and found additional enlarged nodes in the region. She referred me for a biopsy, but the surgeon proclaimed me "young and fit" and sent me on my way. "Come back in a month if it's still bothering you," he instructed, confident he wouldn't be seeing me again. A month passed and the nodes were still swollen. He told me the same thing over and over again. It wasn't until month three that I insisted on a biopsy. After groggily coming out of surgery, I was told the results could take up to two weeks to come back.

The biopsy fell in between Rosh HaShanah and Yom Kippur. My wait for the results overlapped with the *Aseret Y'mei T'shuvah*, the Ten Days of Repentance, when Jews all over the world contemplate their own mortality and bargain with God for another year of life, of health, of snuggles with our children, and of warm days in the sun. On Yom

Kippur I sat alone in the back of a large synagogue social hall reading the words *On Rosh HaShanah it is written and on Yom Kippur it is sealed. Who shall live and who shall die?* I finally understood the meaning of the term "trembling before God." The harshness and finality of the words and the theme of the day offered no comfort, and my anxiety spiral continued.

I had been calling the surgeon's office daily asking for any update, but none had come. Around two and a half weeks post-biopsy I missed the surgeon's call on a Friday at five in the evening. I played his voicemail and heard three terrifying words: "You have cancer." *Who shall live and who shall die?* I frantically called back. The office was closed. The on-call doctor could not help me. This was "not an emergency." I needed to follow up with an oncologist.

The weeks that followed brought a blur of scans, blood tests, and consultations with doctors; sleepless nights on Google preceded hazy days going through the motions of work and caring for small children. I had a false diagnosis of a more aggressive and difficult-to-treat cancer and other scares about scan results in different parts of my body that turned out to be nothing. Until then, I had mistakenly assumed that cancer and its treatment were black and white. Either you have it or you don't; you get treated and are either cured or not. I quickly learned that there is nothing certain about cancer and that it can come with many more questions and subjective decisions than clear directives. With a chronic, rather than acute, cancer whose course of treatment includes "watch and wait," oncologists are much more comfortable with uncertainty. Rather than following a road laid out for me, I had to carve my own winding path.

Finally, I had a diagnosis. A world-class oncologist became a spiritual, as well as medical, lifeline. We crafted a treatment plan. I would undergo radiation therapy with the hopes of slowing or even stopping progression, with minimal side effects. The night before my first treatment, I held my baby girl in my arms, nursing her for the last time, out of precaution. I felt defeated, lost, and angry. This was not the way life was supposed to go. I was only twenty-nine years old. My career, my family, and my life were all just starting. I couldn't imagine living out the future I had planned with the cloud of chronic cancer hanging over everything I did. How much time would this treatment buy me? How many more "last times" would be in the future for me and my precious young family? I remember scrolling that night through my Instagram feed looking at images of all my happy peers smiling with their new babies and feeling jealous; I resented them for their carefree, curated photos. I envied the way I imagined they obliviously enjoyed their adorable children without calculating the expiration date of their time together. I let myself wallow in self-pity and anger. My nascent rabbinate had prepared me for certain situations, but not this.

The next day as I changed into a hospital gown for my first treatment, I felt an urge to pray. I knew about the prayer of gratitude after overcoming a dangerous situation. But what about at the beginning of a dangerous situation, when there was no "overcoming" in sight? I immediately thought of *T'filat HaDerech*, the Traveler's Prayer: "May it be Your will, our God and God of our ancestors, that You lead us in peace and help us reach our destination safely, joyfully, and peacefully. May You protect us on our leaving and on our return, and rescue us from any harm, and may You bless the work of our hands, and may our deeds merit honor for You. Praise to You, Adonai, Protector of Israel."[1]

As I pulled up the Hebrew prayer on my phone in the hospital changing room, its rhythmic cadence soothed me. Its repetition of the word *shalom*—peace—felt like a mantra. Since diagnosis, I had felt utterly alone. Disease seems to have a way of othering and singling out the person who is sick. I had a great support system, but at the end of the day, it was just me in my flawed body. It was my cells alone that woke up one day and decided to stage a revolt against me. In that cold, barren treatment room, it would be just me and the giant, loud radioactive laser so strong that the technicians must take refuge within a lead and metal booth. But, in the changing room, I prayed in the plural: *tatzideinu, tadricheinu, tatzileinu*—lead **us**, guide **us**, rescue **us**. The collective language of our prayer connected me to all the wayfarers of my people, from ancient times through the present.

Baruch atah, Adonai, shomei-a t'filah, "Blessed are You, Eternal, who listens to prayer." The prayer's last line sealed the blessing with a familiar and comforting formula and connected me to all those who cried out to God before and will do so after me—in trauma, in the uncertainty of journeying, in fear, in anticipation . . . and in hope.

T'filat HaDerech sustained me through weeks of radiation, through many checkups and episodes of "scanxiety," and throughout the sacred gift of years of uneventful remission. It is a familiar friend to this day. It reframed my cancer for what it was—a winding journey, not a clear destination—and I was a traveler, not a helpless patient.

A quote attributed to Gilda Radner says that if it weren't for all the downsides, everyone would want cancer. For me, the journey began with extreme beauty and extreme ugliness. The universe revealed its unlimited generosity and expansiveness at the exact same time it revealed its cruelty, randomness, and finite nature. New friends I had just started spending time with immediately morphed into family. They showed up for me in ways that exceeded any expectation, letting me cry to them, bringing me meals, and even writing a song to perform for my medical team at my last treatment (heavily featuring the F-word and requiring the staff to close the doors to the children's wing!). I discovered an online community of "CLL [Chronic Lymphocytic Leukemia] Warriors"—young people living with the same chronic cancer I have, which is almost always diagnosed in old age. Navigating the surreal pain, confusion, and even dark humor of being our doctors' youngest patients broke down any sense of aloneness. As we lost some of our friends along the way, we shared the fear of not knowing who was next, a burden too heavy for any of us to carry alone. Living with a looming threat made ordinary moments with my children ethereal and precious. The rounding of a cheek, a squeal of laughter—the smallest of things that all parents treasure—were suddenly transcendent for me, resplendent and tragic at once. I was gifted a hyper-awareness of the tension between the beauty of how much life has to offer and how quickly it can all be taken away.

With time, the intensity of this awareness has faded. When I find myself bogged down and defeated by normal, everyday stresses, I am both disappointed in myself (have you learned nothing!) and giddy with the luxury of normalcy. I make myself remember a time when I would have done anything for my greatest struggle to be an annoying email or a tight deadline. *Who shall live and who shall die?* I am a different person than the young woman who sat alone trembling in temple on Yom

Kippur, reciting these words while awaiting a cancer diagnosis. I am now much more focused on the end of that prayer: *But repentance, prayer, and righteousness can temper the severe decree.* I am less focused on the when of life and death and more focused on what happens on the journey. It took a lot of time and therapy to get there, and some things can immediately transport me back to the most narrow and scary of mindsets. I know that my journey with cancer is not over and the lessons I have learned will be tested. But, when even the most severe divine decrees can be tempered, when things that seemed fixed reveal themselves to be ever-changing, I make myself view any challenge as a journey rather than a sentence. And I ask the God who listens to prayers for leadership, guidance, and protection along the way.

NOTE

1. This translation is from *Mishkan T'filah: A Reform Siddur*, ed. Rabbi Elyse D. Frishman (CCAR Press, 2007), 114, which is slightly different from the traditional Hebrew prayer referenced by the author.

7

Spoons and Scripture

How Chronic Illness Became My Torah

RABBI ANNIE VILLARREAL-BELFORD, PSYD

I REMEMBER with crystal clarity my first "aha!" moment when study-ing Torah. It didn't come in a Torah or *Tanach* class at Hebrew Union College–Jewish Institute of Religion or while attending a con-gregational Torah study. It came at a Union for Reform Judaism adult learning retreat in 2004 when I was selling books as a URJ Press intern. In between bookselling and quickly eating meals, I was able to attend a class or two taught by Rabbi Lawrence Kushner. I'd consumed many of Rabbi Kushner's books and heard him speak a couple of times, but I had never sat in on a class. He was teaching Torah, and I was excited.

Months before, I had a conversation with a member at the synagogue where I served as an intern. "Annie," he said, "what do we do with those Torah passages that are filled with violence? The ones that talk about killing all the men and taking the women? It is so hard to read those." I replied with all the confidence of a fifth-year rabbinical student and said, "I think we have to consider those passages as remnants from an earlier era. They don't apply to us." It was a tidy—and if I am being honest, dismissive—answer. Those passages exist, sure, but we can just focus on the fun stuff, the easy stuff, the meaningful stuff. I didn't realize at the time, but this was how I approached most of the things in my life: Ignore the bad, focus on the good, move on. This all began to change, I realize now, when I raised my hand in Rabbi Kushner's class.

"Rabbi Kushner," I began, asking about a troubling Torah passage he had just reviewed, "why don't we just dismiss these passages? They are remnants of an era that no longer applies to us." Oh, the chutzpah! Of course, Rabbi Kushner saw right through me. It felt like he gathered the force of every rabbi who had ever taught Torah and grew in stature the way Gandalf does when warning Frodo Baggins about the power of the One Ring in *The Fellowship of the Rings*. In a thunderous voice, Rabbi

Kushner said, "Never assume you know more than the Torah." I was dumbstruck. He later came to apologize in case he embarrassed me, but he hadn't. Instead, his words opened a revelatory new approach to Torah—and to life—that I would learn I desperately needed.

The thing about chronic illness is that there really isn't a starting place. Sometimes chronic illness is like a Rube Goldberg machine, with every symptom and challenge leading helpfully to an end point. More often it is like a scavenger hunt with bad clues and skipped steps. When I started writing this chapter, I thought my first clue was a bad cold that turned into viral meningitis, which in turn led to fifteen months of daily migraines and clinical depression. But by the time I was ready to write the last word, I learned that the migraines—and the cold, and even the meningitis—were just me noticing clues in the middle of my chronic illness scavenger hunt. The first clue was probably the way I walked as a child—toe first, shuffling along, hesitant to fully raise my feet off the ground. Or maybe it was the awkward way I held my pencil, earning my one and only elementary school "Unsatisfactory," in handwriting. A powerful clue was the first time my patella dislocated, something that continued regularly for three years until I had surgery at sixteen. It could have been the dozens of sprained ankles, seven of which led to fractures, eventually also necessitating tendon-repair surgery. It was the acid reflux and menstrual problems, the migraines and the achy joints, the anemia and bloating. In the end, it took over forty years to find the right doctor to look at each and every symptom, read the map of their clues, and diagnose me with hypermobile Ehlers-Danlos syndrome.

Ehlers-Danlos syndrome (EDS) is a genetic connective tissue disorder that affects nearly every system in the body, since connective tissue is everywhere. There are many different types of EDS, with different impacts on the body, and I am relatively lucky to have a milder presentation that doesn't impact my vascular system. Still, I have a constellation of issues that can finally be explained with one diagnosis, something that has brought relief, direction, and tremendous support.

I could enumerate the dozens of small and large traumas that occurred along the way: The emergency room doctor who, after finding out I was rabbi, started to "confess" his lack of attendance at church rather than accurately diagnosing viral meningitis. The doctor who told me that if I lost weight I wouldn't have dizzy spells. The physical traumas of so many injuries to my body. The emotional impact of missing so many important events in my children's lives because I could not get out of bed. The frustration of seeing my life become more and more limited. The persistent suspicion that I was crazy, that everything was just in my head. Chronic illness is a series of ongoing traumas. It robs us of so much—autonomy, energy, trust in our own bodies—and places us at the mercy of a medical system that is siloed, ignorant, and all too often causes more harm than good, especially for folks with any kind of marginalized identity.

But on my better days I manage a gentler approach. For example, I am grateful for a lengthy diagnosis process because I learned so many coping mechanisms along the way. I already had a freezer full of ice packs for my achy joints and headaches. I already had a pillow system (and I do mean system!) to support my body as I slept. Perhaps the most helpful coping mechanism I learned was the "spoon theory," a concept developed by Christine Miserandino to explain the lived experience of chronic illness.[1]

Spoon theory frames one's energy as an allotment of spoons. Getting out of bed and getting dressed requires a "spoon." Going to work when I served in a congregation required five or six daily spoons. Taking care of my kids was a dozen spoons, at least. Some days I woke up and seemed to have all the spoons I needed, but many days I woke up with just a couple of spoons, and it was all I could do to get my kids to school and send an "I am out sick" email to my coworkers before crawling back into bed. Spoon theory has taught me to be more compassionate toward myself and others, to understand that everyone—regardless of their health—has a certain allotment of spoons each day, and to know that many of us must be very thoughtful about the ways we expend our energy.

And on my best days, I am grateful for the illness and its symptoms. I call myself a recovering perfectionist and codependent, and I would never have been able to find the strength to embrace imperfection, deep self-care, and radical self-compassion if I had not gotten so sick. Like many traumas, chronic illness has a way of distilling one's life to its most essential elements, and I released so much that was unhelpful or harmful. My life is challenging, sure—but it is so much better than it used to be.

On an even deeper level, I have turned to my body as a Great Teacher—akin to the Torah. I spent decades ignoring my body or brushing off the parts of it that I didn't like. I used to believe that I should focus on my mind and my soul and that I could dismiss or ignore not just the challenging parts of my body, but my entire body itself. Oh, what hubris! Eventually, I realized that the way I approached my body was like my younger self's approach to Torah, so I learned to apply Rabbi Kushner's words—"Never assume you know more than the Torah"—to my body. Now, my body is my teacher, my rabbi, my Torah. My body always knows the way, even if my brain is slower to figure things out. Today, I see my body as a perfect whole. It rarely does what many other bodies do, but amazingly I love my body now in a way I never could have imagined even a decade ago. There are challenges and there are blessings, but my body—with its aches and pains, its loose joints and stretchy skin, its fat and under-eye circles, its migraines and gut issues—is nothing short of amazing for being able to teach me, guide me, and gently hold my heart and spirit as I experience the physical world.

Pirkei Avot 5:26 tells us that we should "turn it, and turn it, for everything is in it." It is speaking of the Torah, of course, and I think it delivers a message similar to Rabbi Kushner's. I've found this approach applies equally well to how I relate to my body. In fact, the entire *perek* (chapter) applies to how I relate to my body—how we can all relate to our bodies and their conditions—healthy or ill, pained or pain-free, perfect all: "Ben Bag Bag says: Turn it and continue to turn it, for everything is in it; look deeply in it; grow old and gray over it, and do not stir from it, for you can have no better portion than it."[1] Amen, Ben Bag Bag. Amen.

NOTES

1. Christine Miserandino, "The Spoon Theory," *But You Don't Look Sick* (blog), 2003, https://butyoudontlooksick.com/articles/written-by-christine/the-spoon-theory/.

2. Translation adapted from Rabbi Shmuly Yanklowitz, *Pirkei Avot: A Social Justice Commentary* (CCAR Press, 2018), 362.

8

Finding Light Amid the Fractures

Spiritual Lessons from a Bike Accident

RABBI DANIEL B. GROPPER

IT HAD BEEN too many years off the bike. There were years of rabbinical school in Los Angeles and New York and years of parenting children. This and more made going on a long bike ride feel like an entitlement. So I decided to put a damper on the long rides. But cycling allowed me to clear my head, to see the world, to get in a great workout, and to satisfy my love of "techie" things. So one summer, the timing finally felt right. Each ride I pushed a little further. On July 19, 2016—just an ordinary Tuesday, a rabbi's day off—I chose a longer route. Little did I know it would change my life. That morning I dropped my son at day camp and headed out. While on a road with no shoulder, I suddenly experienced a wall bearing down on me. A truck had struck me from behind. Luckily, the only bodily injury was a broken femur. But the accident broke more than just a bone—it broke open a part of my soul.

After waking from the surgery to repair my femur, the rabbi who stood over my hospital bed put it as starkly as anyone could: "You could have died!" It is not how I would have approached a pastoral visit, but he was right—I could have died.

During the weeks that followed, those words rang in my ears. I heard them repeated in different forms: "Boy, you're lucky," "It could've been so much worse," and echoing from within my very being, "I could have died."

A friend who came to see me said, "You're like Jacob, wrenched at the hip bone." Honestly, I was a lot like Jacob.[1] I never stole anything the way he stole his brother's birthright or blessing, but like Jacob, I was arrogant. I felt I was entitled to all I had and believed that others were there to cater to my needs and wants. Humility was not part of my identity. As a congregational rabbi, I had become accustomed to praise and accolades. They became like a drug. I had lost count of how many bet mitzvah[2] and weddings were followed by words of admiration and gratitude. I had internalized all the praises that had been heaped on me over the years and believed that I was greater than I really was. If my dislocation was going to transform me the way Jacob was transformed into Israel, then like Jacob, my path would also take time. If anything, the humility that comes with the idea that "you could have died" became a powerful lesson.

The surgery was quick; the recovery was long and painful. Physical therapy was a long process. The emotional recovery was harder. First, there was the trauma of the accident itself—trauma that uncovered deeper traumas I had long suppressed. I found myself sobbing uncontrollably at the hint of sadness in a movie. I was exploding angrily over the smallest slight. People, especially my family, were looking at me and saying, "He is *not* okay."

I described what was happening to a few people, and they suggested a form of therapy called eye movement desensitization and reprocessing (EMDR). I found a wonderful therapist, and together we unpacked the car accident and an earlier accident during college that caused me physical damage. We unpacked my parents' divorce and my sister's death. She suggested I lean on the power of ritual, so I crafted a ritual for the first anniversary of the accident. I went back to the scene, took a bicycle inner tube, and wrote the words of Psalm 140:8 on it: "You protect my head on the day of battle." I lashed it around the guardrail and reflected on how fortunate I was to be alive.

As this was happening, other things—things about my inner being—also came to light. It became clear that my arrogance had become a huge problem for me and for the people in my life. I was prone to bursts of anger, to communicating in an emotionally cutting way, and—worst of all—I didn't see myself as part of the problem. It was something a caring lay leader pointed out to me when he bluntly said, "You know what I don't hear? I don't hear any contrition from you." I realized that my relationships needed healing.

I started to work with a life coach who guided me in daily meditation with the objective of helping me to become more mindful and equanimous. I learned to practice patience and curiosity, traits that can lead to increased humility. I worked on really listening and went from seeing myself as a victim to seeing myself as someone with agency. Without even noticing, I had become hard and blind to the experiences of those around me; I needed to learn to see others again. I needed to learn to see again. Period.

Living in a world of instant gratification, we look for instant solutions to our problems, but growing in awareness takes time. I continued meditating. I continued reflecting with my coach. I worked really hard on listening, noticing, paying attention to the cues around me, creating more space between stimulus and response. It was hard. It was like flexing a muscle that had never been exercised. Every time I told my coach that I was exhausted or that my head hurt, she responded, "Good, it means it's working."

This coach had me register for the Clergy Leadership Program with the Institute for Jewish Spirituality. It was, to extend the metaphor, an eye-opening experience. For someone who had long eschewed those programs as "woo-woo," I was like a horse to water. I loved the silence of the retreat, the mindful eating, the opportunity to meditate for long periods of time, to practice yoga, to take long walks. I cried copious tears during our worship services. I met a friend and *chavruta* with whom I could be honest and vulnerable. I felt like I was being reborn. The bicycle accident may have broken my femur, but this experience felt like my soul was being cracked open. It felt like the part of me that is naturally loving, curious, and compassionate was breaking through. As the hymn "Amazing Grace" puts it, "[I] was blind, but now I [am beginning to] see."

And then, in January 2019, I had an experience that, after almost three years of hard work, showed me I had really found my sight again.

While on a three-month sabbatical from my congregation, I participated in a weeklong Outward Bound course where, with strangers who would become like family, I canoed down the Rio Grande and slept under the stars. I chose to do this to prove that after a physical setback, I was still strong, capable, resilient, resourceful, and whole. What really opened my eyes was an experience on the last day that led me to a totally new understanding of what "seeing" was really all about.

Overlooking Mexico, I rappelled down an eighty-five-foot rock wall, then began the climb back up. It was easy at first. The handholds and footholds were clear and present. But as I got within ten feet of the top, I froze. "What's wrong?" asked my instructor. I replied, "There aren't any holds. I can't see a way forward."

"What are you going to do about it?" he asked. I realized there were only two options: figure out a way up or rappel back down and live with the emotions of not having made it. I heard myself say, "I don't know what to do. I'm scared. I'm stuck. And I don't see a way forward." Instead of trying to soothe or comfort or fix it, he said, "I want you to try something. Close your eyes." "What!?" came my shocked reply. He continued, "Listen. I've got you. You're not going to fall. Trust yourself. Close your eyes and take a few deep breaths." So I did—seventy-five feet above the Rio Grande, holding onto a rock wall. I took a few slow, deep breaths, centered myself, and then opened my eyes. "What do you see?" he asked. "I see a way!" And I climbed those last ten feet to the summit. Those handholds didn't suddenly appear in the rock—they were there all along. What changed was my ability to see them. In my impatience to get to the summit as fast as I could, and in my arrogance in believing that I knew how to conquer that wall, I failed to see what was always in front of me. The wall humbled me. It asked me to slow down and see things differently. Only by admitting my inadequacy, becoming vulnerable, and asking for help was I able to find a way. To find my way to the top I had to find something that was there all along. To find it, I had to be willing to see things differently.

Of course, just because you see other people, yourself, and your life differently doesn't mean others see the transformation. We tend to create lasting impressions on other people from our earliest introductions. Seeing others in a new light, giving them space to change, and forgiving their past missteps and misgivings isn't easy. I imagine that after that nightlong wrestling match with his newly acquired limp and the blessing of a new name, it still took Jacob's family a long time to see him in a new light, even if he saw himself differently. If anything, proving my internal change to others was going to take more work on my end. I had to deeply commit to my practices of meditation, active listening, experiencing curiosity, and cultivating mindfulness. I had to admit my inadequacies and be vulnerable. And I had to be willing to forgive myself and others on a regular basis.

But just when you think you're almost there, something comes along and hits you like a two-by-four. I was feeling strong and settled, and the feedback I was getting from others was positive. And then the question arrived in an email, "Rabbi, have you forgiven the driver of the truck that hit you?"

All I could think was, "What kind of question is that!? Have I forgiven the driver!? I was the victim! If anything, the driver should be asking me for forgiveness!" Still, I wondered what it would mean to forgive the driver—not to forget the accident, not to release the driver from his negligence, but to forgive—to stop carrying around the hurt and somehow put it down. What would that look like? What would that feel like?

I did a deep dive into books on forgiveness and repentance. I read Maimonides, Simon Wiesenthal's *The Sunflower*, Dr. Louis Newman's *Repentance*, Dr. Harriet Lerner's *Why Won't You Apologize?*, and the work of Everett Worthington, an experienced, respected leader in the emerging field of forgiveness practice. I came to understand that even if the driver of the truck could not ask me for forgiveness (as doing so in a litigious society is an admission of guilt), and despite the fact that it is not a Jewish value to forgive without first being asked, I can still be the one to let down the hurt. I realized that resentment was like carrying around a red-hot rock with the intention of someday throwing it back at the one who hurt me.

The traditional bedtime *Sh'ma* includes the following: "Master of the universe, I hereby forgive anyone who angered or antagonized me or who sinned against me . . . whether through speech, deed, thought, or notion."[3] This prayer is a reminder that the power to forgive is in our hands. We have the power to set down that red-hot rock. One of the most significant things the accident taught me—besides being more careful on the road, having really good lighting, traveling on less trafficked roads, and wearing bright clothing—is to not get so worked up all the time, to let go of things like slights, disagreements, grudges, anger, and resentment, and to be more forgiving and understanding.

In the end, I came to accept that forgiveness is a decision about how you want to live. It's taking control of how much power you allow someone else's actions to have over you and how much power you want to have over your own life. It is a mistake to confuse forgiveness with justice, to think that withholding your forgiveness is a form of punishment for the person who hurt you. In fact, the opposite is often true. As the saying goes, "Holding onto anger is like drinking poison and expecting the other person to die." Besides, why let someone else rent space in your head without paying for it?

Since that fateful day in July 2016, I've thought more and more about the rabbi who visited me in the hospital room. Maybe instead of a rabbi, he was really the angel of death coming to mourn his loss. When he said, "You could have died," he was really saying, "You could have been mine." But I didn't die. I lived. I'm here. I cheated the angel of death, and now I get to say, "You didn't get me. Not this time. Choosing how to live I defeat you over and over and over again!" That's really the key to living in the aftermath of such an accident—we know that we are but a hair's breadth from death and, despite everything, choose to live. How do we choose to live? I choose to live by practicing mindfulness, stillness, and reflection; by breathing, forgiving, and serving; by acting humbly, with vulnerability and curiosity; by being truly human, the way God wants us to be.

Maybe I was like Jacob in that my hip was wrenched and broken—and for a while, so was my spirit. But now, I want to be like Israel—not "one who wrestles with God," as that name is traditionally understood, but one who is *yashar El*, "straight with God"—living my truth and living with a sense of awe for all that is. I keep that thought, and all the lessons I learned, even when I am biking—and living—on this world's crooked, bumpy, accident-prone roads.

NOTES

1. Jacob, the son of Isaac and Rebekah, was a pivotal figure in the Bible. He was known for his cunning nature, famously deceiving his father to receive his brother Esau's birthright and blessing. Jacob fled after angering Esau and spent years working for his uncle Laban, eventually marrying Laban's daughters Rachel and Leah. He fathered twelve sons, who became the heads of the twelve tribes of Israel. Before entering Canaan after a twenty-year absence, he had an all-night wrestling match with an unnamed being, who wrenched his femur at the hip bone. Jacob's life was marked by struggle, transformation, and divine encounters, culminating in a reconciliation with Esau before his death.

2. Bet mitzvah is a gender-inclusive term for the Jewish coming-of-age ceremony.
3. Translation adapted from *The Complete Artscroll Siddur: Nusach Ashkenaz* (Mesorah Publications, 1990), 289.

9
Hawks and Snakes and Not Giving Up

Rabbi Robert A. Nosanchuk

A RABBINIC PARABLE tells of a dove who, fleeing an avenging hawk, hides in the cleft of a rock. There she discovers a vicious snake! The presence of the snake makes her safety impossible. The hawk draws closer. What does she do? She screams. She flaps her wings! She is Israel fleeing the Egyptians, who could not enter the sea, for it had not yet split. Nor could they retreat, as Pharaoh would kill them. What did they do? They admitted their fears and cried aloud. They were redeemed (*Shir HaShirim Rabbah* 2:14:2).[1]

Jewish history is filled with stories of our people fleeing predatory hawks and dangerous snakes. Exodus teaches us that what saves us is admitting fear. Screaming is not giving up. Flapping your wings is a way of demanding no one give up on you. Generations have found this parable relevant to the struggle to run faster than real and metaphorical predators that pursue us.

Rabbis regularly see key components of this midrash realized in congregant experiences. Still, over my thirty-plus years of service in the community, a singular threat most resembles the parable above: cancer! This disease has been called the "emperor of maladies" by physician and author Siddhartha Mukherjee. He explains this appellation's basis in Job 18:14, *melech balahot* (king of terrors). Rabbis used to be further removed from such terror, acting primarily as educators and adjudicators. But contemporary rabbis are included in the constellation of caregivers witnessing how cancer or adverse effects of its treatment wound the bodies and terrorize the spirits of the people we are pastoring. We encounter people realizing there is no hiding space. We hear them scream and see them "flap their wings."

A twelve-year-old preparing for her bat mitzvah confessed her fear that cancer would kill her mom. Her fears were legitimate; her mom died on the operating table days after celebrating the family milestone. It's been twenty years since I told her that her mom died. But I still hear echoes of her wailing in that waiting room. She grew to be an accomplished divinity student at the graduate level. However, she also became afflicted and passed away from complications of a different disease. As a rabbi still in the life of her father and brother, my role is to hold space for their alternating rage and fear. It's been critical to not ascribe meaning as to why disease strikes. This helps push back against a perception among some Jews that their rabbi is akin to an attorney on God's "defense team." Instead, I try to convey that rabbis are among those who can prosecute a substantive case against the unfairness of a daughter losing her mom and then a father losing his daughter. Rabbis can do our best work in gentle empathetic expressions of concern shared with families touched by diseases such as cancer.

To me, holding space also means not being visibly rattled when witnessing a distressed person or their loved one react to a terribly unfair circumstance. It is isolating to be diagnosed with something that may not kill you now, but could in the future. Hawks begin to circle above. While rabbis should stay out of game plans for medical treatment, those afflicted with cancer often need their spiritual leaders to pay attention to the chaos taking over their lives and help sort through it without judgment. What I've found is that people fighting cancer often ask me if I'll help them "go to war" with God or whomever they perceive as dealing them such a monstrously awful hand.

In April 2019, the notion of cancer as a monstrous hand dealt to people became very personal. On the last day of that month, I learned that a predatory cancer secretly attacked and was metastasizing within me as stage IV melanoma. My case originated from an unknown location. Due to its fast-spreading nature, I sprinted into oncological care.

Before my diagnosis, I'd been a "man with a plan." I was packed for a flight to Israel, and my suitcase was in the car. I was jetting off from Cleveland to guide dozens of congregants touring Israel. Several days after my return was my child's planned bet mitzvah. It was ambitious. But I had felt empowered to plan for so much professionally and personally.

At midday of April 30, 2019, every ounce of my empowerment drained from me. Hawks began to chase. A Cleveland Clinic oncologist explained the severe danger of the cancer stalking me. I grew at once terrified and also terribly hopeful. Just a few weeks earlier, a CT scan following unrelated abdominal pain showed a suspicious mass near my adrenal glands. This required scans, ultrasounds, and a needle biopsy. Had I ignored my pain or had my doctors lacked vigilance, no doubt I'd have no time to fight. I also recognize that the medical profession, even if it means well, took my abdominal pain seriously and scrutinized it with more swift attention than is often done for women and other marginalized communities.

A couple of days after my Israel trip, I began infusions of checkpoint inhibitor medications, the most potent form of cancer-fighting immunotherapy. The record related to such medicines taming cancer was only a few years old, yet data on their effect was much more promising than any other option. This was my very best shot at survival, at least in the near term. I remained determined to take each and every one of the twenty-four monthly infusions, even though my body suffered multiple adverse effects.

That is probably why, even after learning of the severity of my cancer diagnosis, I still traveled to Israel on that planned trip. I believed this could be my last trip anywhere. But I have sometimes regretted that I didn't find a way to set my work aside and instead go somewhere with my spouse, Joanie, where she and I could work on developing the hope, positivity, love, and strength we needed—and continue to need—for my fight and my comeback.

For other worthy reasons, we left plans in place and decided to temporarily keep my diagnosis a secret. I guided my trip, returned home, and began treatment immediately before our child's bet mitzvah. We felt that if cancer was as ferocious as we'd been warned, we wouldn't want to have our last major family event seen through the perspective of tragedy and heartbreak. And . . . our plan worked . . . almost.

Late evening of the bet mitzvah Shabbat, adverse effects from my first infusion grew rapidly. I was terrified and traumatized and soon quarantined in the hospital. There I began to call family members expecting to see me at a family brunch and instead tell them I was in a big fight and needed their help. This was, in effect, my version of the dove crying out for help, and the encouragement, hope, and presence of loved ones became essential to me as I managed two more hospitalizations that summer, at a time when it was unclear if treatment was having anything but disastrous effects. My first scans began to show some minimal progress . . . but progress nonetheless!

Midway through my two-year course of immunotherapy, doctors indicated it was safe to operate and remove the cancer site. Fourteen treatments later, my scans were stable; at the end of treatment, they were free of metastasis. It is now five years since diagnosis, which was almost an inconceivable milestone before the discovery of immuno-therapy treatment and the availability of checkpoint inhibitor medica-tions. My cancer has been declared in remission. I am truly thrilled!

But "thrilled" doesn't describe all I feel. While it is true that cut-ting-edge treatment saved my life from a predatory disease, the adverse effects of my cancer treatment itself nearly killed me. What tamed my cancer also left my body inflamed, my mind scorched, and my spirit wounded. Denying this does me no good. I'm on the run again, but this time what I'm running for is not safety from harm. Rather I'm running toward improved brain health, cardiac health, mental health, and spiri-tual wellness. I've needed to cry out for help. But in addition to doctors and therapists offering medical interventions and rehabilitation strat-egies, I've now got the prayerful intentions of my temple members in my corner.

A huge asset to my getting my spirit and attitude in the right frame was my childhood rabbi, Dannel Schwartz, z"l, who—more than any-one in my life—got in my face when I needed it and also held my hand when that's what he perceived would help. He took turns between those modes of rabbinical caregiving while the toxicity of my treatments and the inflammation they caused grew. During two years of active treatment, there were many cries and the occasional instinct to run away from it all. Paramount to my comeback and helping my mindset was the comforting presence and support of my childhood rabbi. We always offered one another God's honest truth. During one of our times together, I confessed to him that, in a way, my body and spirit as I knew them before cancer had already died. Cancer treatment killed what had once been intellectually facile brain power and decayed my body's mus-cle mass. My fingertips—which used to be able to sense my surround-ings—are nothing but numb, due to neuropathy. I felt like a part of me died when I listed for him the activities that are no longer achievable. I spilled out these confessions to my rabbi at lunch a little over a year ago when my wife stepped away from the table. He listened to me carefully. Then he watched me take the medication that mitigates the inflammation in my body from cancer treatment. I spilled out all my concerns and he didn't step back, become repelled, or give me advice. He leaned in and placed his hand on my shoulder. He told me, "I want you to live." He praised my work at rebuilding to achieve a new peak in my physical and mental health. Together we agreed that if my worst fear arises and cancer does come back, what I'll need most is strength and speed with which to chase cancer back to its hiding place.

It is of little surprise that a health crisis caused me to struggle both physically and spiritually. Rabbis aren't immune in any way from having faith tested by forces abusing our bodies and spirits. Before diagnosis, I could never relate to people who'd concluded they must've done something to deserve their struggle with cancer. I now relate precisely to that fear! For no matter how potent a medicine one takes, internal doubts of my own self-worth kill with just as much cruelty as metastasizing cells. I'm on a positive trajectory. But in my loneliest moments, I do wonder whether I am worth the fight.

Dr. Rachel Naomi Remen writes about spiritual experiences within the realm of her own caregiving as a physician. In a Facebook post, she recalls a time when she personally received anesthesia for a medical procedure. Just before sedation, the surgeon asked if he might say a prayer. When she assented, the doctor whispered, "Dear God, help us to do here whatever is most right." Upon hearing her surgeon's prayer, Dr. Remen says she felt "release" from an "almost paralyzing fear that had been my daily companion."[2]

My own cancer experience has changed the way I relate to congregants yearning to have something release them from the fearful place where the mind of a cancer patient dwells. Learning that I had cancer with enough time left to fight it, I've been blessed to be able to declare a permanent "before" and "after" marker in my life. My "after" has thus far eluded the grip of cancer recurrence. I haven't died yet. So I try to be like Dr. Remen's surgeon, a caregiving presence who prays for and promises and delivers what is "most right" to people I encounter. This soothes my spirit. But as a person who also struggles with self-worth, I believe that in some small way, this activity ennobles the commitments I have yet to make in life. Yes, I dread the idea that metastatic disease will recur. But until that time or some other eventual harshness afflicts me, the most critical care I need at this stage in my life can't be infused into my veins. I need human empathy, understanding, and acceptance of the path I travel.

These qualities have been essential since early in my treatment, when my oncologist began to express growing concern that my cancer medications were possibly killing my colon. We fought over my next steps. She didn't want me to underestimate the challenges of potentially living out the rest of my life with a colostomy bag attached to me. But she also empathized and listened to me with understanding. She respected me when I explained that if a potential-emergent colitis delayed my infusions and gave melanoma time to keep spreading, I'd blame myself. We struck a deal that broke our impasse, and I continued to go on with my infusions unabated.

I've since had to negotiate deals with doctors strategizing with me over treating lasting effects of treatment—neuropathy in my toes and fingers, loss of thyroid function, joint inflammation, and neurocognitive deficits. Just a few months before I concluded treatment, it also became clear that cancer had severely damaged my adrenal glands' ability to produce cortisol. Ironically, we need adequate cortisol to boost our energies, particularly when facing a threat to our lives! Cortisol helps us quickly take flight from danger or recover from wounds. Now I permanently take medicines to replace dangerously low cortisol. This way, I won't die because some other factor than cancer weakened me or put me in danger. My medicine and my strengthening mental health will help me fight or take flight if necessary. I don't minimize the combination of medical and mental health interventions I need. My body needs reinvigoration, but so too do my soul and spirit.

I use daily mindfulness meditation, communal prayers, and rituals as tools in that soul strengthening. I have begun to use acupuncture as well. There are times when I'm reflecting quietly on my situation while in an acupuncture treatment, when I realize how blessed I am to have been among those whose names have been prayed in multiple faith communities, all conveying their highest intentions for my well-being.

Shortly after my diagnosis became public, a man from my temple was waiting by my car for me at the end of my workday. A friend with kids of a similar age, he playfully called out my name as I exited the building like I was a player being announced as the next pitcher to run in from the bullpen. I hadn't called him to ask him to come by. He hadn't told me he was coming, and he never mentioned cancer. He had just received the email from our temple notifying him about my illness, and he decided to just show up. As I got closer, he opened his big arms and wrapped them around me and whispered in my ear, "I've got you." Several weeks later, a dear friend and leader in the Muslim community called me to insist that each day ahead, I should taste a small spoonful of honey. He explained this instruction comes from a teaching about expansiveness and healing within the Qur'an. He wasn't trying to convert me to Islam or foolishly trying to convince me that honey cures cancer. What he wanted from me is not to withdraw from experiencing that which sweetens life. I learned here, and not for the first time, that illness can create the opportunity to bring us closer to people and closer to stories not our own.

It is more than reasonable to doubt the effects of hope, solidarity, or sweetness to buoy a person fighting a predator such as cancer. I am as skeptical as anyone about what the will of another person's love can do to protect someone from a growing tumor, fast-spreading metastasis, a dangerous medical complication, or a sudden cancer recurrence. But there is a strengthening effect that comes from others holding you in the light of their prayerful optimism.

If forced to go "on the run" from cancer again, if what lies ahead is a sea that hasn't yet split and what chases me is a killer disease, I hope I'll believe in redemption and choose the sea. As a rabbi, I've seen too many people taken from their families at critical life moments, and I don't want to share their fate. For all I know, the roughest part of my struggle is complete, or the worst may still lie ahead. But cancer's terror doesn't go away. It hovers near, awakening internal anxieties. I don't dwell on it, yet I also can't ignore the substantial possibility of recurrence. Still, I am determined not to give up. I won't give up on hope, nor will I give up on redemption. I may scream. I'll certainly flap my wings. But I won't give up. I'll ask God to hear my screams as a plea for help or a sign of life. If there is a God, the Holy One could take notice and help me receive the attention I need to help me heal. If there is no God, I'll have to trust that my help can come from doctors and researchers, counselors and rabbis, all doing and acting on "what is most right."

NOTES

1. Interpretive translation by the author.
2. Rachel Naomi Remen's Facebook page, accessed September 29, 2014, https://www.facebook.com/rachelnaomiremen/posts/10152751758294882/.

10

The Next Chapter

Moving Forward with Chronic Illness

RABBI DAVID N. JAFFE

Opening

AS I LAY THERE in the darkness, I was left with nothing but my thoughts and the continued beeping of the infusion pump by my side. It was 3:00 a.m., and as usual, the infusion pump read "patient occlusion." This was my third night in the hospital and the third night in a row that my thoughts were accompanied by the beeping of the infusion pump. My thoughts and feelings were overwhelming. My fear and shock had turned to anger and confusion. I had just been diagnosed with a severe case of ulcerative colitis, an autoimmune disease that is a chronic illness. For the first time in a while, I had a strong desire to do something—anything. It was the first time I felt any type of motivation to move or act, and I decided I wanted to pray. But how? And what? My mind began to race. There I was, a fifth-year rabbinical student, a lover of Jewish liturgy, sick and lying in a hospital bed, and I wanted to pray, but I didn't know what to pray.

Initially, I thought I could say *Mi Shebeirach*, our prayer for those who are sick, and simply add in my own name at the appropriate time. Yet, in *Mi Shebeirach* we pray so that God may cause our "health to be restored" and for God to grant us "a complete renewal of body."[1] I was processing what it means to have a chronic illness, and I knew that it was with me forever. My health could not be "restored," nor could I achieve a "complete renewal of body." This prayer didn't work for me. Next, I thought about *Birkat HaGomeil*, our prayer for surviving a traumatic experience. I had certainly done that. But was my traumatic experience behind me? I was still lying in a hospital bed. I thought about the words of *Birkat HaGomeil* and its praise of God for goodness being bestowed upon us. I felt many things in that moment, but gratitude for the goodness God bestowed upon me unfortunately was not one of them. This prayer, too, would not suffice. So, what did I pray? I didn't.

The next day came, and I had my mother bring me a siddur so I could further examine our liturgy. I hoped I would find something I could connect with. When I opened *Mishkan T'filah* for my morning prayers, I didn't make it past the first line of the first blessing. The opening line of *Asher Yatzar* reads, "Praise to You, Adonai, our God, Sovereign of the universe, who formed the human body with skill, creating the body's many pathways and openings."[2]

Again, I felt alienated. I was newly diagnosed with a disease where my body misinterprets information and mistakenly attacks itself. In *Asher Yatzar* we praise God for creating the human body with skill and wisdom, yet my body was attacking itself! Did God mess up? Did God just make an oopsie? *Asher Yatzar* is a blessing praising God's miracles and ability to heal all flesh, yet my autoimmune disease would never be cured. I felt lost, scared, and isolated.

This was the first experience of many more to come that emphasized I was different. From this moment forward, my life would have two very distinct chapters: "pre-diagnosis" and "post-diagnosis."

Chaos and *Keva*

The experiences described above took place during the months of July and August of 2021, immediately before the start of my fifth year of rabbinical school at Hebrew Union College–Jewish Institute of Religion (HUC-JIR) in Cincinnati. Over the course of the next year and a half, I would have three hospital stays, would try four different types of medication therapy that all failed, see three registered dietitians and four different gastroenterologists, work with two different therapists, and receive more blood tests, CT scans, and ultrasounds than I can remember. Lest I forget, I would also finish my fifth year of rabbinical school, become ordained as a rabbi, have over twenty interviews throughout the rabbinic job search, get married, move across the country, and start a new job. My life at the time could be summed up in one word—chaos. It was a period that felt like a roller coaster that stretches high into the sky, only to drop me and let gravity do its thing. I felt as if there was no stopping and no navigating. Everything felt out of my control. It was as if my life was a Jackson Pollock painting. I began searching for something, anything, that would help bring a sense of stability to my life. My help came in the form of prayer—not in the specific words of the prayers, but the ritual act of praying.

In Jewish prayer, two concepts are generally discussed: *keva* and *kavanah*. In the context of prayer, neither *keva* or *kavanah* is easy to translate, as their meaning exceeds a simple one-word parallel in English.

Kavanah is an absolutely vital element of Jewish prayer. It has been said that "prayer without *kavanah* is like a body without a soul."[3] *Kavanah* can be understood as intention, attention, inwardness, direction or directing oneself, and even true spontaneity. I sometimes like to understand *kavanah* as follows: Imagine a situation where someone has a deep desire within them. They act upon this desire. Their actions and their thoughts are in perfect alignment and harmony. *Kavanah* is the inspiration and motivation that caused the person to act. *Kavanah* is us, at our most vulnerable moments, acting upon our innermost desires.

In the prayer context, *keva* can be understood as our "fixed" liturgy or our routine prayers. *Keva* is our tradition. Professor and scholar Jakob J. Petuchowski states that *keva* represents the constant found in Jewish prayer all over the world. Petuchowski writes, "This need for a recognizable constant leads to the gradual crystallization of fixed parts of the worship service which remain, with very minor local modifications, always and everywhere the same. Thus a prayer tradition comes into existence, a routine element which gives community worship its 'fixed' aspect. It is what the ancient Rabbis called *keva*, the fixed, the routine, the traditional."[4] *Keva* provides a foundation upon which we can stand and rely. Because *keva*, by its very nature and name, is fixed, constant, unyielding, and stable, the *keva* in our prayer structure is reliable.

As mentioned earlier, the months around my diagnosis were utter chaos. *Kavanah* comes with a sense of spontaneity and requires one to be fully invested in the moment. In my moments of trauma and chaos, spontaneity was not something I needed, and being fully present in my moment was not something I wanted. Rather, I wanted some control—something that I could rely upon amid the randomness. Thankfully, Judaism and its complexities and plethora of practices offered me a powerful tool to create stability in my life: *keva*.

In Jewish practice (with the exception of the lighting of the Shabbat candles), it is obligatory to bless before we act. For example, when we raise the *Kiddush* cup on Shabbat, we say a blessing and then drink the wine. When my life turned to chaos, I began to recite blessings before all of my actions. Before brushing my teeth, I would recite a blessing. Before taking a walk, I would recite a blessing. Before entering a classroom to learn, I would recite a blessing. Before listening to music, I would recite a blessing. This, I learned, was the power of *keva*. By reciting a blessing before an action, regardless of the specific words that I might be saying in that blessing, I was creating something reliable in my life. I had some control. The *process* of *keva* provided structure and reliability when my world was random and unpredictable. Additionally, I felt great comfort in engaging with a Jewish practice—reciting a blessing prior to acting—that had spanned millennia. Those three to five seconds of saying a blessing before acting was a catalyst toward the acceptance of my disease.

I do want to stress that these blessings were not blessings of healing. There was no "Oh God, heal me and provide miracles so that my illness will be gone!" No—chronic illness does not work that way. Instead, I prayed to pray. I learned that no matter what happened in my life, I could always pray. This was my *keva*.

A Box and a Soul

Abraham Ibn Ezra was the epitome of a Renaissance man. He was born in approximately 1090 in modern-day Spain and is known today for his commentary on the Torah and his linguistic bravado. Ibn Ezra writes in his book *Y'sod Mora V'Sod Torah* (A foundation of awe and secret of Torah) about the use of words and language. Ibn Ezra describes each word as having two parts: a *teivah* and a *nefesh*. The *teivah* is the "box" in which the word is presented, and a *nefesh* is the "soul or being"—the true meaning of the word that is hidden inside. Every single word, he claims, comes in a fancy box (*teivah*), but what is important is the word's meaning, its *nefesh*. While Ibn Ezra spoke of words containing a *nefesh* and a *teivah*, so too do human beings have these components. Each one of us has a *nefesh*, an inner true self that only we know, that only we experience, and a *teivah*, a box that we present to the world. When our *teivah* and *nefesh* don't reflect each other, it can feel terrible. There can be deep inner pain that no one can see.

For those who are chronically ill, it is common to present a *teivah* of strength while our *nefesh* is in pain. We are a part of what Meghan O'Rourke calls an "invisible kingdom." She writes, "The more I talked to sick people, the more I found that what is most disturbing for many of us is that grace has become a kind of moral requirement in sickness."[5]

In the middle of my chaotic experience was the interview process for becoming a rabbi at a congregation. Throughout the interview process, I felt I had to present a *teivah* of strength, bravery, and grace, while my *nefesh* was in pain. In one such interview for the position of assistant rabbi at a large congregation, I was asked what Jewish ritual I found most meaningful. I responded with *HaMotzi*, our prayer for eating bread. To my surprise, dismay, and a bit of embarrassment, everyone on the Zoom screen laughed. One person said, "Well that was unexpected! We haven't heard that one before!" Reflecting back, I do not hold anything against those people who chuckled at my response of *HaMotzi*. After all, Judaism is filled with numerous important rituals that mark and shape a lifetime. The people on the search committee with whom I shared my response had no idea that I spent weeks without eating solid food, lying in a hospital bed grieving the loss of the life I had imagined, attempting to accept my new reality, and longing for the moment when my doctor said I could eat solid food again. They didn't know how much I yearned to say *HaMotzi*. They also didn't know how meaningful a moment it was for me when I finally could say those words over my plain, soggy hospital toast. I pray that you never know just how delicious and joyous hospital toast can be.

Thanks to Ibn Ezra's teaching, I learned that we see others' *teivah*, the box they present to the world, and not their *nefesh*, their inner self. I began to seek the *nefesh* in other people, and with that came empathy and compassion. I was slower to judge others based on the *teivah* they were presenting. With a greater sense of empathy and compassion toward others, I began to finally be compassionate toward myself.

Closing

There is another prayer concept that is important to note—minyan. A minyan is a group of ten individuals coming together to engage in Jewish prayer. There are some prayers, like the Mourner's *Kaddish*, that in traditional spaces require the presence of a minyan. Essentially, one idea behind this requirement is that when people are at their most vulnerable, such as after experiencing the loss of a family member, a group of people is necessary to help them make it through the stages of grief. When we are experiencing trauma, our community can help us. You don't need to go through trauma alone. While generally the obligation to form a minyan falls on the community rather than the suffering individual, the person suffering has to allow them to help. I learned that asking for help was not a sign of weakness, but a sign of strength.

On July 31, 2021, I was diagnosed with a severe case of ulcerative colitis. We often use language like "moving on" or "just let it go" when it comes to trauma, yet my illness is something that is lifelong. I can't "let it go." Thankfully, Jewish practices have enabled me to move forward in my life *alongside* my illness and have helped me seek acceptance. This trauma will forever be with me, and still Judaism has helped me find comfort, stability, and compassion within my trauma.

Notes

1. Translation from *Mishkan T'filah: A Reform Siddur* (New York: CCAR Press, 2007), 109.
2. Translation from *Mishkan T'filah*, 32.
3. Don Isaac Abravanel, *Yeshu'oth Meshiḥo* (Jerusalem, 1967), 14a.
4. Jakob J. Petuchowski, *Understanding Jewish Prayer* (Ktav, 1972), 7.
5. Meghan O'Rourke, *The Invisible Kingdom: Reimagining Chronic Illness* (Riverhead Books, 2022), 261.

11

Discovering Holiness

A Jewish Love Story in the Shadow of Alzheimer's

RABBI DEBRA R. HACHEN

IT'S ALMOST 11:00 A.M. and I sit in my living room gazing across the valley at the hills that divide Walnut Creek from Alamo, California. Just over that hill is a home where Peter, my husband of forty-five years, is ten years into living with Alzheimer's disease. As his wife, I live it with him.

It began in New Jersey. At age sixty, Peter was let go unexpectedly from his dream job as chief technology officer for a Jewish nonprofit. In retrospect, his declining performance was due to undiagnosed mild cognitive impairment. Once he was home full-time, I could see all was not right. I attributed it to depression and anger at the job loss. My first true inkling of Peter's dementia was at a restaurant when he said he could not calculate tips. I remember exactly where I was sitting. It was the first of hundreds of small shocks that burned themselves into my memory. There is a drawer in my brain with ten years' worth of snapshots or soundbites of such moments: a phone call that he is lost in the rain on a street corner in Manhattan, a wastebasket thrown down the garbage chute with the trash, a critical document fed into the shredder instead of the copier. We saw none of that coming that night at the restaurant, but I must have sensed the possibility.

Three years later everyone around Peter knew he was struggling. He knew too.[1] Each person with Alzheimer's disease progresses differently and with varying symptoms. In these first years, Peter lost more than his ability to understand numbers. He could not do tasks with more than two steps (loss of executive function). He lost words and names though he still knew the person or object in front of him (expressive aphasia). This man, who once wired a friend's speakers and installed programs on computers, now could not keep track of passwords or use a spreadsheet.

In the fall of 2014, when our doctor in New Jersey first wrote "possible dementia" in Peter's chart, I had no idea what it meant to be the wife of a husband with Alzheimer's disease. It took my breath away. Still, my first thoughts were: I am strong, I am a problem solver, I can handle this. Navigating the convoluted medical system soon taught me the truth about dementia journeys. Nothing is easily managed.

In the spring of 2015, after numerous physical tests ruled out other causes of his dementia, Peter drove us to the daylong neuropsychology testing. He was now sixty-three years old. After only two hours, the psychologist cut the tests short. Peter's dementia was too severe. A report would follow, but Peter should stop driving immediately. He took out his keys and handed them to me.

That small gesture was typical of Peter's characteristic gracious acceptance of what later was confirmed as Alzheimer's disease.[2] It was also confirmation that more and more of the previously shared duties in our marriage were becoming my responsibility. I could not control this disease, but I had to be ready for it. Some preparation was easy. I found support groups for us both. I did my research and shared it with him. Knowing the years were limited, I began planning trips from our "bucket list." I arranged updated legal documents.

It was the little things that began to overwhelm me. With the stress of diagnosis completed, anxiety caused by hyper-alertness moved front and center. I was constantly on the lookout for signs of his decline so I could create a workaround. It was like whack-a-mole. Adjust, adjust, adjust. Manage, manage, manage. The fixes could be simple but the quantity—and the time they consumed—increased over the months, then years. One week, he needed me to point out the sock drawer. Soon, I had to lay out his clothes on the bed. Later, I had to hand them to him one at a time. His losses were my gains—in the worst possible way. Every task he could not handle moved to my to-do list.

"It must be so hard for you," friends would say to me. "Yes, but it's harder for Peter," I would shrug. After all, he was losing his ability to navigate the world independently. He was losing the normal dreams of a man in his early sixties with grown children—looking forward to weddings, grandchildren, and more. He hated the moments of brain fog and confusion.

At the same time, there was goodness in his life. He had me and a circle of family and friends he trusted completely to watch over him. He was easygoing and outgoing. His own father had died when Peter was just sixteen, so he never counted on his life being a long one.[3] Peter's mother had dementia at the end of her life, so his diagnosis did not surprise him. Yes, it was very hard for him when his brain failed him, but he embraced the challenge in a very Jewish way.

All his life Peter had been dedicated to the Jewish values of social justice and *tikkun olam* (repairing the world). He looked upon his disease as an opportunity to make a difference. Rather than hiding his disease, he had a passion for explaining it to others. He hoped this would make life easier for someone else. It gave him purpose.

Meanwhile my focus remained on the everyday hardships and keeping my head above water. I was strapped into a front-row seat for his decline. Each time his life shifted, mine did too. He was losing pieces of himself, and I was losing him. I was losing the husband who supported me, comforted me, challenged me, laughed with me, mourned with me, and knew me in a way no one else ever would. I was losing the love of my life, who caught my eye and gave me a wink each Friday night when I looked out from the bimah. There is a name for this experience: ambiguous loss. "Ambiguous loss is a type of loss you feel when a person with dementia is physically here, but may not be mentally or emotionally present in the same way as before."[4] In dementia's cruel twist, the less Peter was "with" me emotionally, the more he was physically present in my life. We moved through the world even more as a couple, but I was feeling more and more alone.

In 2016 I started a list on my computer of Peter's inabilities. They were coming fast and furious. Can't make coffee. Forgot how to use an ATM. Ate cereal with a fork. Started to shave in the middle of the night. I wanted a record to share with his doctors, family, and friends. I hoped tracking his illness would prepare me for what was to come.

One day as I skimmed the list preparing to record another incident, a switch flipped. What was I doing? Alzheimer's disease was relentless. The list of what he could no longer do would inevitably grow longer. I saw that recording his losses was objectifying him. It was a way to hold him and his illness at arm's length, to hold back the grief growing inside me. Was this what I wanted to do for the years we had left? Would this lessen the pain when he became fully incapacitated and inevitably died?

With one click, I created a new list. This one enumerated his wonderful qualities, the things that made him happiest, and how he contributed to our family and the world. Peter ushered at the temple. Peter laughed at puns. Peter loved a good glass of scotch with friends. Peter kayaked and hiked and told great stories. I started looking to create more moments like that for us both. I tried to take pleasure in the simple things we shared and be grateful while they remained. I didn't want to lose the Peter I loved—a multifaceted person who did not deserve to be defined by his deficits.

Peter and I resonated deeply with the teaching that each person is created *b'tzelem Elohim* (in God's image)—capable of goodness, kindness, and justice. As I now paid closer attention to the beautiful image of God in Peter, I was in awe of the grace with which he lived with his dementia.

Yes, Peter was more than his disease, but what was I? Could I think of myself as more than a wife responding to the ravages of her husband's disease? Could I live more gracefully even though I was already anticipating his death,[5] unable to name all my losses, and anxious about what was coming next?

I could see the strength in Peter, but not always in myself. Others would admiringly tell me how brave and attentive I was, how lucky Peter was to have me as his wife. That's not how I usually felt. I felt I was doing what was required of me. If I appeared brave, it was because Peter needed stability. If I was attentive, it was because that was how I kept crises at bay. Many turned to me for advice about dementia because I seemed to know so much and explain it so well. At those times I put on my rabbi hat but often felt like a fake. Underneath I felt so inadequate. I didn't want to become an expert; I wanted to lean on experts. Mostly I just wanted to put my head under my pillow and block out the world. That was not an option.

Though I had become adept at seeing the image of God in Peter— reminding myself to be patient and kind toward this soul bound up in a declining body—I was not taking care of my own soul. I needed to nourish my spirit so we could continue to truly be "soulmates."

Around this time, I began attending a support group for spouses my age whose partners had dementia. They had similar misgivings and regrets, failures and successes. We trusted each other because we walked the same path. We could laugh at the foibles of our loved ones and rant about this disease. They helped me envision what was coming. I began to feel brave, competent, and strong.

The time finally came when Peter could no longer be left alone. Friends would help, but I knew the time was close when I would need to retire to be with him full-time. Being a congregational rabbi had been central to my identity for nearly forty years, but we had always put our marriage first. On Peter's sixty-sixth birthday in the summer of 2017, we met with his neurologist. I needed her professional advice about the anticipated speed of his decline. Could I work another year? I wanted to be living near our middle daughter in California for support when Peter reached the last stages of this disease. When would be a good time to move? She replied, "Tomorrow." She urged us to do this while Peter could still adjust to a new place and new people.

With both sadness and relief, I gave my notice to the congregation that night. No one was surprised. In the fall, I drove us cross-country to our new home. In many ways, we had a lovely first year. We welcomed our first grandchildren. I found a new support group. Peter made some new friends. We found three Jewish communities to explore on Shabbat. It was such a joy to sit side by side holding hands during the services. Peter's years as a rabbinic spouse meant that he had numerous melodies and Hebrew prayers on the tip of his tongue. We could lean against each other during the *Mi Shebeirach* (healing prayer) and stand together holding hands during our parents' *yahrzeits*. The sanctuaries truly provided sanctuary that first year in California. They were a safe, familiar place, but also holy space. There, I could let go of the declines and challenges and let the rabbis and cantors watch over us and carry us along. When I was a pulpit rabbi, new congregants would often share that they came on Shabbat for community more than prayer. I was there for both—to pour out my heart in prayer and to forge bonds that might connect me to community when Peter was gone.

Those restful hours at Shabbat services were meaningful but fleeting. A little over a year after our move, Peter needed me with him constantly.

He shadowed me in every room. He paced if left with anyone else. He needed assistance with eating, toileting, and dressing. I was up numerous times in the night to guide him back and forth from the bathroom. I was sleep deprived, depleted, and burned-out from doing three eight-hour shifts daily. A man in my support group reminded me, "Anyone can be a caregiver, but only you can be his wife." I knew it was time to do what Peter and I had agreed upon years earlier. He moved to a memory care unit and called it his second home.

Now a team did the caregiving. Peter was the youngest resident, and the staff loved him. I did the fun things. I took him out a few times a week for meals, walks, and visits with friends. We attended some Friday evening services and a wonderful informal Shabbat morning service from time to time. For a year we found a new balance. While Peter's body and mind were steadily weakening, mine were growing stronger as I recovered from being constantly "on."

Then came COVID. All visitors were banned. I was afraid Peter would not get the individual attention he needed, would forget me, or would die of the virus. I felt helpless and anxious. Each Friday I would drop off a challah at the front door, and the staff would connect us on Zoom later in the afternoon so I could sing Shabbat blessings with him. He found the Zoom confusing and soon could barely mouth the first words of prayers. By the time we were reunited a full year later, he had lost his last words and had to be propped up in a wheelchair.[6] In the fall of 2021, it was clear Peter needed a smaller, quieter environment, and I moved him to the nearby small care home. These last two years, despite being bedridden, Peter seems comfortable and content.

This quieter period of his illness has given me time to "practice" moving through the world on my own, in preparation for when Peter is truly gone. I have chosen one of the congregations as my Jewish home and been warmly accepted as a congregant and as a retired rabbi. I choose activities and friends carefully, saying no to situations that I now know might trigger stress. I am still recovering. I live every day with anticipatory grief by my side and am not sure what I will feel when he dies. I do know that others will be there to embrace me when that time comes.

Most days I sit by his bed talking to Peter for an hour or so. Music he used to enjoy plays in the background. He often stares at the ceiling or falls back asleep. I might feed him his lunch or dinner. On Fridays, I sing his favorite Shabbat songs. I hold his hand while we listen to Debbie Friedman's *Mi Shebeirach*. I no longer focus on the second verse that asks for physical and spiritual healing. Instead, my mantra has become the line "Help us find the courage to make our lives a blessing." I now believe those who told me how brave I was. I do believe that the *tzelem Elohim* within me, my presence and love, have been a blessing in Peter's life. When the prayer finishes, I often speak to Peter about the numerous ways that his life too has been a blessing. Sometimes he looks me in the eye, and I wonder what he sees.

I know what I see. I see the gentle man who trusted me with his dignity, safety, and happiness. I see the husband who let me love him through it all and never stopped loving me in return. I see the soul behind his beautiful eyes, where his spark is waiting to be released. I want to hold onto it, but I know I will eventually have to let it go. I hope I will be ready.

NOTES

1. Many with Alzheimer's disease have anosognosia; they do not understand they have dementia. Peter was spared that symptom.
2. Peter had a PET scan that was definitive for Alzheimer's disease. Later, a genetic test unsurprisingly showed he was a carrier of two alleles for APOe4, which indicates a 70 percent chance of developing Alzheimer's.
3. On our first date he warned me that the men on his father's side had all died young of heart problems. His father had lived the longest, to his mid-fifties.
4. "Ambiguous Loss and Grief in Dementia," Alzheimer's Society of Canada, 2019, https://alzheimer.ca/sites/default/files/documents/ambiguous-loss-and-grief_for-individuals-and-families.pdf.
5. Anticipatory grief is grieving before the loved one dies. With dementia, that can be many years of grieving without closure.
6. Three years later a doctor surmised that Peter had developed Parkinson's disease in addition to his Alzheimer's. This also ran in his family.

PART THREE

Trauma of Marginalization

12

Calling Out to God

Trauma and Transition

RABBI ARIEL TOVLEV

AT FIRST, "transgender" was a thought experiment, a curious lens with which to shift perspective. I did not seriously consider the possibility when one summer day I languidly asked my college boyfriend, "What would you do if I transitioned?"

Without thought he responded, "I would break up with you."

A small jolt ran through my veins, and the conversation no longer felt theoretical. "Really? You wouldn't even try?"

He shrugged.

It was not sadness I felt at the time; I did not yet have any idea that I was trans. But the emotion took over my body: My skin went clammy, my jaw clenched, my body contracted, my heart hardened. What I felt was fear.

Once awakened, the fear found a home in my body. It churned my stomach, stayed my tongue, and made me question myself. *What if no one will love me?*

Coming out did not quash the fear. It surreptitiously spread throughout my body, gradually growing stronger. Every stranger staring, every family member questioning, every friend with passing advice, every politician dedicated to destroying me, every micro- and macroaggression fed my fear.

"It's such a shame you will never pass as a man. You have such a feminine face."

"It's not possible to be transgender and Jewish. Transgenderism goes against the Torah. You have to pick one."

"No one understands 'nonbinary.' You should just say you're a trans man."

"I'm bisexual, but I like men to be men and women to be women. I'm not attracted to trans people. It's just my preference."

"You were such a pretty girl. Why did you give all that up? Is it worth it?"

"We don't offer transgender health care. Transgenderism goes against our religious beliefs."

"Transgender people using bathrooms that go against their biological sex are deviants and predators, and we need to protect our children."

Like a web spun throughout my body, like mold spores scattered and multiplied, like a root system taking hold, eventually there was no spot free from the fear.

Unknown to me, the compounded trauma was being stored in my soul not as sadness, but rather as fear. Fear disguises itself as rational, protective, and transformational. Fear told me I could be safer. Fear told me it'd get better if only *I* changed; everything was in my control because everything was my fault. My fear became my guiding force: As long as I was vigilant, I could prevail.

I struggled to connect to my own sadness while fear had its hold on me. Jewish tradition has prescribed times for sadness: sometimes for just a moment, like with the Mourner's *Kaddish*, a prayer recited daily in remembrance of those who have died; sometimes for a portion of a day, like the *Yizkor* (Remembrance) service held on Yom Kippur, Sh'mini Atzeret, Passover, and Shavuot; and only once for a whole day, on Tishah B'Av, the day we mourn horrific losses in Jewish history. On Tishah B'Av we are meant to fast, dress as mourners, sit on the floor, and read Lamentations—a Biblical book about the destruction of the Temple and the devastation that followed. One Tishah B'Av, attempting to dive into the morose mood of the day, my best friend and I were reading Lamentations. Amid the despair and utter hopelessness, this line stood out to me: "Of what should a living human complain? Each of their own sins" (Lamentations 3:39).

This is the truth, I thought. *Our life is a gift. Nothing else is guaranteed. We cannot expect safety, comfort, or love. As long as we are alive, God has given us all we are owed.*

Only now do I realize that was my fear speaking. On a day meant for mourning, I couldn't feel the loss in Lamentations. To feel loss, I'd have to let my walls down. I'd have to allow my heart to break open. I'd have to be vulnerable. But vulnerability is incompatible with vigilance.

Fear disguises itself as rational, protective, and transformational. My fear transformed me. While my transition started as a way to express my most authentic self, my fear told me I would never be accepted as nonbinary and should live as a trans man. I accepted the lesser of two untruths to survive. I changed myself to fit what people expected from a transgender person. I stopped sharing that I was nonbinary, even with close friends. I stopped believing that anyone would want to understand the real me. At one point I noticed that despite being surrounded by people, I had never felt so alone. I had to consider: Is it better to be in community living as someone else or to be alone living as yourself?

"From a narrow place I called out to God, and from an expansive place God answered me. God is on my side, I have no fear; what can a human do to me?" (Psalm 118:5–6).[1]

I felt trapped, trapped in a narrow place. The narrow place—*hameitzar*—shares the same root as *Mitzrayim* (Egypt). The place where we are enslaved. The place where we live without God. The place where we cannot experience freedom. From the narrow place, I turned my sight to the expansive place, the place of liberation and salvation.

I turned to God for help. Over and over, I called out, each cry bringing glimmers of clarity. It was not instantaneous, but like puzzle pieces coming together, I received my answer: I may have been pushed into a crevice through others' invalidations, but I had the power to free myself. I recalled the story of the famous Chasidic rabbi Zusya, who said, "In the world-to-come, they will not ask me: Why were you not Moses? They will ask me: Why were you not Zusya?"[2] Instantaneously my fear shifted, and I felt like Zusya: Instead of being afraid of disappointing others by not meeting their expectations, I became afraid of disappointing God by not living authentically as the unique creation They intended.

Everything changed so quickly. The expansive place provided an entirely different perspective. I was meant to be different, and my difference was a gift from God. As I fell in love with myself in all my wholeness, I also wholly fell in love with the person who is now my spouse. I embraced my own gender queerness as I embraced my spouse's. I found my voice. Poetry poured out of me. The complex fabric of fear woven into my bones started to disintegrate, evaporating like a shallow stream in the summer sun. *Leave this narrow place*, I told myself. *Go to the expansive place. God is with you. What can a human do to you?*

As it turns out, humans can do a lot.

I was thirty-two years old when I was sexually assaulted by a medical professional. I had just moved, found a new doctor, and made an appointment to refill my testosterone prescription. The doctor didn't understand what being transgender meant. As I was trying to explain it to her, she became increasingly frustrated. Rather than asking additional questions, she put her hand in my pants and felt my genitals.

I felt that terrifying jolt of fear in my veins once again. All the interweaving fibers that had dissolved over the years ignited and solidified. A flash flood of fear coursed through me; it took only a second until my body became unbearably heavy, weighed down with webs long forgotten but not lost.

A familiar voice entered my head. *You don't deserve to be treated like a human being. You are an object, an oddity, a body without a category.*

The doctor took her hand out of my pants, relieved with understanding.

"Okay, you're a woman," she concluded. She went to her computer and changed my documentation to "female," undoing all my work fighting for a male gender marker.

"Anyway, we don't prescribe hormones here," she continued. "You're going to have to go to a gynecologist."

It would be two years before I saw a doctor again.

Despite prior success freeing myself from my fear, it was not easy to replicate. I went right back to that narrow place, feeling like no one could hurt me if no one could touch me. My walls came up, a fortress against vulnerability. I couldn't feel sadness; sadness would mean admitting that I was wronged, that I deserved better, that the world is cruel and I was a victim of it. No, fear felt safer. Everything was in my control; I was safe as long as I was vigilant, as long as I closed myself off physically and emotionally.

God could not answer me because I did not cry out.

Years went by. I dove into our prescribed moments of sadness: *Yiz-kor*, Tishah B'Av. Once again, I could feel sadness only for others. For myself, only numbness.

For many, trauma may exhibit itself as sadness. It may materialize like a stone in one's stomach and grow to become an immovable weight. Some of my external trauma—such as the death of my good friend at only thirty years old—did function like this, forming a pit of loss and despair. But my personal trauma became fear. To connect to my own despair, I had to first comb through the webs of fear and coax my soul out of the narrow place.

I know you are hurt. I know you are scared. You deserved better. Do not hide any longer. Come out to the expansive place, where you can be with God again. Come out to the expansive place, where you can feel the warmth of love and joy. Your narrow place is not a shelter; it is a prison. The expanse is vulnerable, but it is the only way to truly live. Come out, come out. I love you.

From a narrow place, a crack within a cliffside, squeezed so tightly I could barely tell where I ended and the rock face began, I let a small cry escape my lips. For so long I had been silent out of fear of being found. I could not be silent any longer.

Oh God, please help. I'm alone and afraid. I don't know where to go from here.

I am with you, the sunshine said as it squeezed through the cracks to rest on my shoulders. *I am with you*, the breeze said as it brushed against my back. *I am with you*, the trees said as they rustled their leaves in encouragement. *I am with you*, the ground said as it shot forth sprouts, preparing padding for my fall. *I am with you*, my heart said, pounding with anticipation.

What can a human do to me? I cannot list all the threats. There are endless ways to be abused. I am full of fear. Sometimes I feel like I am nothing but fear. But God is on my side.

As long as I call out, God answers:
Come out, come out. I love you.

Notes

1. Translated by the author.
2. Martin Buber, *Tales of the Hasidim* (Schocken Books, 1991), 251.

13

Alcoholics, Addicts, and Finding Ourselves in Judaism

RABBI SUSAN B. STONE

THERE ARE LOTS of people who don't drink alcohol. But when someone can tell you that it has been forty-one years, nine months, and four days (at the time of writing), chances are that person who is keeping count is not some casual teetotaler. Chances are that person (me) is a recovering alcoholic.

The details of how I got here are hardly fascinating and, in fact, are of a time and place that does not reflect today's reality for addicts and alcoholics.[1] What I share with these individuals is that something I once believed was the answer to my life's problems ended up becoming the biggest problem in my life. Even when it became clear that my drinking was causing issues, I still wanted to keep it in my life, hoping that I could make it a solution again.

My choice for sobriety came as the result of a crisis. In many ways, my life got better just because I was no longer under the influence. But it was far from that miraculous solution I once thought alcohol and other drugs provided. As with many alcoholics, I had a host of problems to address in my early recovery. In terms of my sense of self, shame was at the top of the list. But that was hardly all. The wreckage of my past cut a wide swath, and that repair had its own schedule. I found this repair and new solutions with the help in a twelve-step program.[2]

After some years of (re)building my life, I saw that many of the problems fueling my addiction were still there. The sense of spirituality that grew from working the Twelve Steps provided much of that elusive solution I'd been pursuing. But it didn't feel complete until I was able to connect my sober spirituality with my Jewish life. Yes, it is fair to ask, "Why not earlier?"

I did have a fine seminary education, and we are a God-acknowledging people, but incorporating Judaism into my recovery wasn't easy. As my recovery progressed, I began to understand that, to me, spirituality meant I could live a life of purpose, grown from a reality beyond my own making. I needed to grow into that understanding before I could search for Jewish grounding.

I sought teachers, groups, and texts that could offer support, but I confronted both the explicit and embedded structural messages that othered me, and those like me, from the rest of the Jewish community. Examples include the well-known Yiddish refrain *a shikker ist a goy* (a drunk is a gentile) to enduring a seminary professor claim that giving children Shabbat wine inured them against future misuse of alcohol. I had such experiences while I was working to repair my life. Part of that repair was realizing that I also had a particular voice and could challenge the silence that grew from the Jewish communal fear of opening ourselves to gentile derision if Jews were to "air our dirty laundry in public."

I—and many others—did just that.[3] We began by talking to each other. And then we tried talking to our congregations, our institutions, and our fellow Jews. We organized groups and conferences. We wrote. We taught. We preached. We made some headway.[4] Yet the response of the institutional Jewish community was limited and cautious. Many tried to make addiction out to be an "adolescent problem" or only showed interest in addiction recovery if they could monetize the counseling process in Jewish-run agencies rather than embrace Alcoholics Anonymous and other proven programs. This response did not create the bridge between recovery and our religion and offer the help that so many Jews in recovery hoped to find.

The next piece is the most important part of this story. I'll tell you the end first: We Jewish alcoholics and addicts found ourselves in the texts and teachings of our tradition.[5] This was where we began to find the long-desired sense of grounding.

Here are three small examples that made a world of difference:

- We discovered that Purim was also about us. You see, there is a commandment, based on the Babylonian Talmud, *M'gillah* 7b, that one should get drunk on Purim. Specifically, the Rabbis teach that one should get so drunk on Purim they could not

differentiate between "cursed" Haman and "blessed" Morde-
chai. Well, we were the ones who already got so drunk so often
that we couldn't tell blessing from curse when we needed
to. Seeing ourselves and accepting our addiction gave us a
healthy, genuine claim to be part of the Jewish story!

- We discovered that, like Dinah—the daughter of our patriarch Jacob, sister to her twelve brothers—we also had an urge
to roam. The Torah (Genesis 34) describes how Dinah "went
out" from her home to visit her neighbors. Tragically, she
was raped while on her excursion, forced to marry her rapist,
and then witnessed her brothers kill her rapist and his family.
From the innocence of motive, she suffered greatly. But her
family moved heaven and earth to rescue her. Many of us only
wanted our families to come back for us as well.

- We discovered that B'ruriah's voice was respected during a
time when women were rarely valued publicly. B'ruriah—
daughter and wife of respected Rabbinic sages—was known
for being deeply knowledgeable about Torah and Jewish law,
and the Talmud contains multiple stories where her brilliance
is on display (such as in Babylonian Talmud tractates *Avodah
Zarah*, *B'rachot*, and *Eiruvin*). She challenged the norms, and
yet we still honor her. Just like we'd hope for ourselves!

As a rabbi and an alcoholic, I could not best live my life until Jewish
teachings and practices were included in my recovery. As I found many
parts of my story in the traditions and texts that form the basis of our
religious community, the spiritual solution of recovery grew to include
Jewish teachings. That helped heal me. As others have the same opportunity, this solution may help heal our larger community as well. When
we alcoholics and addicts see ourselves in these texts and institutions,
we take our place in the community. We enrich it as it enriches us. As we
acknowledge the connection and others acknowledge us, we all benefit.

We Jews in long-term recovery are people who often construct our
spiritual identities from twelve-step recovery work and then add the
specific words and teachings of our tradition that sustain and enrich
recovery. In this way, we live a hybrid formed of both Jewish and

universal spirituality. Instead of only benefitting us, we believe that this model may allow other Jews in dire straits to find recovery in a similar way—embracing both the wisdom of the general world and the fruits of our tradition. Those of us in recovery see the pains of our community through a particular lens and want to do our unique part to help heal them.[6]

It is necessary to address one last point.

I was hesitant to write this piece because I have been sober for so long. Longevity is no badge of honor or wisdom. In Alcoholics Anonymous, the saying is "All I did was not drink or die." You see, today's context of addiction is different than in years past. As hard as it was for us, it is harder for people to get sober today than it was all those years ago. There are a few reasons for this. First, many drugs today are partially or entirely synthetic. These synthetic components act differently on the brain and the rest of the body, making withdrawal and recovery more difficult. In addition, our profit-driven health-care system serves itself best when medicating patients rather than treating the root causes of their addictions; therefore, some of the issues that may have contributed to addiction may never be addressed, creating a cycle of recovery and relapse. Finally, there is a compassion fatigue crisis among caregivers when it comes to this disease, with ever-increasing rates of relapse. Addiction is a problem that doesn't go away.

But there is always hope. We have more awareness, more acceptance, and a great desire to grow the tent of Jewish life. The Jewish community has received some valuable lifesaving lessons over the forty-plus years since I began recovery.

We've learned that our "protective" actions weren't so helpful and that we have to proactively save lives, rather than rely on shame, fear, and xenophobia to keep us safe. We've learned how to better respond when someone comes forth with their suffering. We've learned to listen without asking intrusive questions. We've learned that it's not just "the kids" who have problems. We've learned that neither money nor zip code confers protection from addiction. We've learned that we can survive and even thrive after heartbreak and challenge.

And we're still learning. We're still wrestling with all our texts and traditions. We don't want recovery to just have a Jewish patina. We want

Judaism to be interwoven with recovery. We still need more proactive engagement, like adult education curricula that address the reality that Jews in addiction and recovery have an impact on all of us.

We're still learning that sometimes it's okay to take a back seat to those who were previously excluded by the organized Jewish world and let them lead us. At its core, the essence of recovery is finding a workable spirituality. For Jews, that has always been found in community. The inevitable God-wrestling will be to everyone's advantage.

For us addicts and alcoholics, we're still learning that those of us in recovery are different but also not really so unusual. Don't treat us as examples—we are your children, your parents, your outcasts, and your leaders.

We're still learning how extensively trauma affects the addict, their whole family, and our community. We need to welcome those exploring Judaism anew as they recover from addiction, and we need to normalize their trauma and find the vocabulary that will allow us all to be at home as Jews.

My first boss was a rabbi of "the old school." He was a brilliant scholar and preacher. He ran an effective congregation and stood with his congregants at the best and worst moments of their lives, providing a steady Jewish context to their days. He knew I was in recovery and didn't care. But there was the day that he gave me a congregant's phone number and asked me to call them for counseling. The background information that he gave me: "They're interested in all that spiritual stuff you're always talking about." I knew I was home.

Notes

1. Throughout this chapter, I will use the terms "alcoholic" and "addict" interchangeably. It is a popular, though not universal, practice. There is both scientific and scholarly debate on this point.

2. Programs such as Alcoholics Anonymous, Narcotics Anonymous, Gamblers Anonymous, and the like are all based on twelve steps. These steps become the foundation for a person's recovery when worked on with a peer (sponsor) and in fellowship with others similarly affected. Similarly, support groups for friends and family members of addicts and alcoholics, such as Al-Anon, Codependents Anonymous, and Nar-Anon, rely on the same twelve steps.

3. I must tip my hat and heart to Rabbis Jim Goodman, Richard Ettelson, Abraham Twersky (z"l), and Rami Shapiro.
4. Two of the early accomplishments that can be celebrated are the JACS (Jewish Alcoholics, Chemically Dependent Persons, and Significant Others) Foundation and the Bay Area Jewish Healing Center.
5. We owe a great debt to feminist and queer pioneers who, when similarly searching for full membership in Jewish life, reexamined our texts and found themselves in them.
6. There is scholarly evidence that intergenerational community trauma contributes to elevated rates of addiction and alcoholism in minority communities. As people who embody this finding, we dare to hope that our recoveries may help those who also bear these afflictions but have escaped the addiction burden.

14

Learning to See in the Dark[1]
A Jewish Approach to Depression

RABBI DEBRA KASSOFF

A person must cross a very, very narrow bridge.
The main rule is: Do not be frightened at all!
—Rabbi Nachman of Bratzlav, Likutei Moharan 2:48:2:7

(In my sleep I dreamed this poem)
Someone I loved once gave me
a box full of darkness.
It took me years to understand
that this, too, was a gift.
—Mary Oliver, "The Uses of Sorrow"[2]

You must judge every person generously.
—Rabbi Nachman of Bratzlav, Likutei Moharan 1:282:1:1[3]

YEARS BEFORE I suffered with major depression, still more years before I learned that Rabbi Nachman of Bratzlav wrote of his own struggles with what closely resembles the condition we now call clinical depression, I loved his teachings.[4]

Years after my diagnosis, after my depression had been treated and (mostly) managed, I learned of Rabbi Nachman's struggles with mental illness and studied his teaching about *n'kudot tovot*, "points of goodness." You must find just a little bit, he taught, even so little as a single point, of goodness in every person. In every person—including yourself. This will enable you to praise God. When I learned this, something substantial shifted in me, like gears falling into place, like the sun falling beneath the horizon, revealing stars.

But I'm getting ahead of myself. First, there was darkness.

I don't remember a lot of specifics from my early bouts of depression, which I experienced as a mental and spiritual darkness. I've noticed throughout my life a tendency to forget many details in general, and the details of negative experiences in particular. I don't hold grudges. I prefer to give people the benefit of the doubt. "Judge everyone generously" comes naturally to me, mostly.

Still, some sensory impressions remain.

What I remember: the feeling of weight. A great weight sat upon my chest, making every breath heavy. Something terrible pressed on my spirit, turning even the most brilliant landscapes, the sweetest experiences, a shade gray, a touch bitter.

I was living in Israel for my first year of rabbinical school. The love of my life, my future husband, had moved to Israel for the year and made plans to study there, just to be near me. I was beginning glorious friendships, finding my people, studying subjects that stirred and challenged me, embarking on the fulfillment of a dream. I was at Judaism's spiritual center, moving daily—even while running errands or cleaning the apartment—among and within ancient holy places.

And yet this heaviness made everything more difficult, from getting out of bed in the morning to appreciating the beauty of a sunny Jerusalem day to completing my school assignments. It covered everything with a gritty pall, a vague but persistent sense of dread.

The depression wasn't completely without context. I had, only a few months before my departure for Israel and the start of rabbinical school, lost a dear friend—a brilliant and beautiful but very broken soul—to suicide, the result of brutal mental illness and deep spiritual wounds. There were rituals of mourning, both religious and secular, along with the support of many loved ones, to help navigate the grief.

But the darkness did not lift with passing months. It persisted. It followed me back to the States. Eventually it was given a name, a diagnosis. And it's been faithful; though responsive, thankfully, to medication, it has never entirely left me. Each time, in the nearly thirty years since, that I have tried—by design or circumstance—to leave pharmaceuticals behind, the depression came crashing back.

There were always triggers—the roller coaster of hormones, emotions, and new challenges following childbirth, a particularly intense period of work stress, or a major life change. Each began by affecting me as it might anyone: with sadness or anxiety. But where others might notice the pressure and the gloom beginning to relent, I repeatedly found myself at the bottom of a pit that held me fast against the forces of time, reason, a return to equanimity, love, or hope. It kept me captive until I resumed both drug and talk therapy.

In these times of pandemic, climate disaster, and war, sometimes—even with a medical buffer—I have felt its tendrils plucking at the edges of my mind, slender legs of darkness threatening to puncture my resilience, to turn the solid ground beneath my feet to shifting rubble.

During my sojourn in Israel, I started along the path of what has become a lifelong interest in the representation of darkness, both literal and figurative, physical and spiritual, in Jewish tradition. When it was my turn to lead a service in the Hebrew Union College–Jewish Institute of Religion chapel on King David Street, I chose darkness as my theme. With my first-year rabbinical student skills, like a treasure hunter wielding a gardener's trowel, I scraped references to darkness out from the soil of Jewish tradition wherever I could find them.

What I found was both plentiful and wonderful. Of course, I encountered a rich vein of sources confirming the light = good / darkness = evil paradigm.[5] This paradigm comes rather naturally to anyone who has ever survived a long night of terror, quaking at the prospect of all the dangers darkness might be hiding: creepy-crawlies, stumbling blocks, would-be assailants, or nightmares. But I also found something else. As I stumbled through my inner darkness, fighting not only the depression itself but also fears of being exposed by its presence as broken or defective, I discovered in Jewish wisdom a different perspective. I encountered a regenerative, creative, redemptive aspect of darkness that gave my experience of depression an entirely different frame.

For example, the midrash teaches, "You find that a person standing in the dark can observe what is transpiring in the light. However, anyone standing in a lighted place is unable to observe what is happening in the dark" (*Midrash Tanchuma, T'tzaveh* 8:1).[6] Another midrash from the same source reads, "Rabbi Berekhiah said: Consider the eyeball. It is not through the white of it that one sees, but through the black. The Holy One, blessed be [God], says: 'If I create light for you out of the darkness, what need have I of your light?'" (*Midrash Tanchuma, B'haalot'cha* 5).[7]

Whether in your own lit home at night, or around a campfire in a nighttime wilderness, or in the Israelite homes during the plague of darkness on the Egyptians—to sit in a place of light where darkness presses all around is a privilege indeed, and a comfort. But it also presents a handicap: We miss everything, nefarious or beautiful, transpiring just beyond our circle of light, in the dark.

As the poet Wendell Berry has written:

> To go in the dark with a light is to know the light.
> To know the dark, go dark.[8]

Paradoxically, a whole new world of vision opens to us when we "go dark." Not only do we see things from darkness, and in darkness, that cannot be seen otherwise, but things happen in darkness that will not happen where the sun shines, literally or figuratively. Life in general, and Jewish tradition in particular, bears this out.

In her commentary to *Parashat Vayeitzei*, Avivah Zornberg notes the sunset at Bethel—so named by Jacob following his dreamtime revelation of God's presence—and the sunrise at Peniel—after his all-night wrestling match with a mysterious stranger who gave him the name Israel—framing the *parashah*. "Between these two points," she writes, "there is darkness, the Dark Night of the Soul."[9] Yet in the crucible of this difficult, materially enriching but spiritually painful twenty-year sojourn with his uncle, the clever but heartless boy who stole from his brother and tricked his father grows into a man who knows God and knows himself—humbled, yet father of a nation, heir to a divine covenant. In darkness, Jacob found God and found himself.

According to the Jewish calendar, when the sky grows dark, a new day begins. According to Jewish tradition, when the sky grows dark, new life begins: "There is an angel in charge of conception," the Talmud teaches, "and his name is Night" (Babylonian Talmud, *Nidah* 16b).[10] This connection between darkness and new life runs deep. From a midrash we learn, "Three creations preceded the world: water, wind, and fire. Water became pregnant and gave birth to darkness" (*Sh'mot Rabbah* 15:22).[11] All life begins in water, requires water. And all new beginnings, new insights, new creations, it seems, require darkness.

"Lean into it," a wise friend in Jerusalem advised me of the depression. "Find what it has to teach you." Having uncovered just the slenderest slice of the vast treasure Jewish wisdom contains on the gifts of darkness, this resource together with my friend's words gave me courage to allow myself simply to be in depression, not to fight it or despise it, not to berate myself for my feelings. Still there were days when I could not imagine relief, when all I felt was a stagnant despair. Still, I required medication to come (and stay) out of it. Yet somehow, it seemed less painful, less terrifying, easier to endure, now that I had permission to sit, watching from my darkness, waiting to see what might be getting ready to be born.

Which brings me back to Rabbi Nachman of Bratzlav. The world is a very narrow bridge, carrying us over an abyss of—of what? Darkness. Chaos. The mysteries that precede and succeed our amazingly brief lives here. One misstep, it seems, might plunge us into the deep, end the journey. A fearful prospect. Yet, paradoxically, fear more than anything makes the way perilous. Meanwhile, the darkness contains gifts. From darkness comes life; from darkness came light.

Some have found Rabbi Nachman's teachings particularly challenging where it comes to the matter of depression: "It is a great mitzvah to always be happy, and to make every effort to determinedly keep depression and gloom at bay."[12] While Rabbi Nachman's teaching nowhere suggests that depression or other sorts of illness are sinful, he does suggest that all illness is the source of gloom and depression. Some have criticized this line of thinking as potentially dangerous.[13]

We now know there is some science behind what Rabbi Nachman intuited. Joy, laughter, releases stress and promotes physical as well as spiritual health. But we also know what Nachman likewise understood implicitly: That which we resist, whether it be darkness, depression, fear, or any other supposedly negative emotion or experience, only becomes larger in our consciousness. That which we accept dissipates.

So: Walk the very narrow bridge (without guardrails, no doubt), but do not fear.[14] How? By accepting the fear. Know that our nature is "to draw itself to gloom and depression," but also that one must "force oneself to be happy at all times." How? Not by fighting the depression, but by "bringing oneself to joy any way one can—even by silliness."[15] Above all, we may dispel the fear, find some happiness, by judging everyone generously—even oneself—and insisting on finding at least a spot of good, of joy, of light, even in the midst of terrible pain and darkness.

We who have sat in the dark have great courage, and great compassion. We have a sensitivity for goodness, and light, and beauty, and joy—precisely because we have walked through places where none could be found. We could still see it, though, still find it. We could manufacture it, "even by silliness," if necessary, and we can see it now a mile away. One develops a great appreciation for that which one once lacked. An appreciation for and sensitivity to even the most modest sources of light and joy—this is a point of goodness indeed.

So now I always imagine Rabbi Nachman of Bratzlav, leading his community in ecstatic communication with the Holy One through singing, dancing, mystical stories, leading them to joy, to God, eyes streaming tears, feeling joy, heart breaking. Each of us carries all the emotions within us. The despair of depression is not wrong. It is not sinful. But as consuming as it can feel, it is also not all of us. We can only find our way through the darkness, find our way to joy, however broken, shot through with sadness, by leaning into it. Knowing how to do this, knowing how to praise God even in the midst of deepest darkness—

> It took me years to understand
> that this, too, was a gift.

A gift that our Torah and Jewish tradition are exquisitely well equipped to teach us.

NOTES

1. The title of this chapter is inspired by Barbara Brown Taylor's *Learning to Walk in the Dark* (HarperOne, 2014). Unless otherwise noted, all translations are by the author.

2. Mary Oliver, "The Uses of Sorrow," in *Thirst: Poems* (Beacon Press, 2006), 52. Reprinted by the permission of The Charlotte Sheedy Literary Agency as agent for the author. Copyright © 2006 by Mary Oliver with permission of Bill Reichblum.

3. Translated by Rabbi Arthur Green, PhD, "The Teachings of Rebbe Nachman" (lecture, informal HUC-JIR alumni retreat, Cape Cod, MA, June 4, 2009).

4. Rabbi Nachman of Bratzlav was the great-grandson of the founder

of Chasidism, the Baal Shem Tov, and was credited with the revitalization of Chasidic Judaism in the late eighteenth century. For details on Rabbi Nachman's mental health diagnosis, see Arthur Green, *Tormented Master: The Life and Spiritual Quest of Rabbi Nahman of Bratslav* (Jewish Lights, 1992); Joseph Weiss, *Mechkarim B'Chasidut Breslav* (Bialik Institute, 1974); Ada Rapaport-Albert, *Chasidim V'Sabata-im, Anashim V'Nashim: Studies in Hasidism, Sabbatianism, and Gender* (Zalman Shazar Institute, 2014); Jay Michaelson, "'Unhappy Happiness,' Or What Rabbi Nachman and Pharell Have in Common," *Forward*, August 16, 2014, https://forward.com/opinion/204199/unhappy-happiness-or-what-rabbi-nachman-and-phare/.

5. Lest we become confused by legitimate concerns about racist assignations of value or lack thereof to people whose skin is characterized by its relative lightness or darkness, I wish to clarify that the light = good / darkness = evil paradigm referenced here precedes and transcends our modern understanding of race. The paradigm, while in my view limited, is not itself morally problematic. The inappropriate way in which racism has transferred our associations with darkness—that is, the absence of physical or spiritual light—to people with melanated skin is what's problematic.

6. Translation from *Midrash Tanhuma-Yelammedenu*, trans. Samuel A. Berman (license: CC-BY-NC, https://creativecommons.org/licenses/by-nc/4.0/), found on Sefaria (sefaria.org).

7. Translation from Hayim Nahman Bialik and Yehoshua Hana Ravnitzky, eds., *The Book of Legends, Sefer Ha-Aggadah: Legends from the Talmud and Midrash*, trans. William G. Braude (Schocken Books, 1992), 87.

8. Wendell Berry, "To Know the Dark," in *Terrapin* (Counterpoint Press, 2014).

9. Avivah Gottlieb Zornberg, *Genesis: The Beginning of Desire* (Doubleday, 1996), 185.

10. Translation adapted from Bialik and Ravnitzky, *The Book of Legends*, 547.

11. Translation adapted from Bialik and Ravnitzky, *The Book of Legends*, 17.

12. Nachman of Bratzlav, *Likutey Moharan*, trans. Moshe Mykoff (Breslov Research Institute, 1986–2012), 2:24:1, found on Sefaria (sefaria.org).

13. Rabbah Atara Cohen, "A Jewish Theology of Depression," *Lehrhaus* (blog), April 26, 2018, https://thelehrhaus.com/scholarship/a-jewish-theology-of-depression/.

14. If every one of us must indeed cross a very narrow bridge, suspended over who knows what, if we accept this metaphor for existence, then it would seem unreasonable—foolish even—to have no fear. Although the plain text does not directly support this, I like to resolve the contradiction by

understanding the phrase *lo l'facheid k'lal*, which is often translated as "do not be frightened at all," as "do not be frightened in general," following the meaning of *k'lal* as "rule." I see Nachman shouting at his students, arms waving, "Of course the world is a scary place! You would be fools not to be frightened! The whole world is a very narrow bridge, terrifying, but the important thing is—do not be consumed by your fear. Do not allow fear to overtake you. You are more than your fear."

15. Nachman of Bratzlav, *Likutei Moharan* 2:24:2:1.

15

T'Mol Shilshom, Reflecting on Times Past

The Trauma of Disability

RABBAH RONA MATLOW, DMIN

I HAVE KNOWN trauma from a very early age, including physical, verbal, and sexual abuse. Ironically, when I left college and enlisted in the Navy, boot camp felt like stress relief.

During my twenty-two years in the Navy, I served on six ships—two submarines, two nuclear cruisers, an anti-submarine frigate, and a repair ship. While I never saw any combat, for which I thank God, I was injured and received permanent disabilities on all but the first submarine. On my last ship, the second nuclear cruiser, the injury was to my neck. This would become the most devastating of my injuries.

In my final assignment, riding a desk, I began to experience numbness and tingling in my left arm. Ironically, my sister was diagnosed with multiple sclerosis (MS) at the same time. It was very unsettling that her symptoms were identical to mine. So, I got an urgent consultation with the neurology department at the military hospital. After anxiously awaiting the results, I was told, "Congratulations, you don't have MS; you have a neck injury!"

I retired from the Navy in pretty good shape, even with the developing neck issues. My wife and I settled in the West Mount Airy neighborhood of Philadelphia in an affordable row house. I stood out as relatively young and fit among our elderly neighbors. I helped them with tasks like shoveling snow and doing repairs. I felt like the block's superhero! Then, in 2005, the neck injury drastically worsened. I started experiencing devastating and radiating neck pain, with numbness and tingling down my arm returning with a vengeance. The pain was debilitating, and suddenly, in a very short period, I went from superhero to living on permanent disability.

I lost a tremendous amount of what previously defined me: my physicality. My mother (of blessed memory) called me her "six-foot bottle opener." I could not serve that role anymore. I couldn't open an empty sauce jar without a helper at that point, I was so weak.

I was dismissed from my chaplaincy residency due to my disabilities. I needed two neck operations and would not have been able to complete the requisite training for the program, so I was removed from it. I was emotionally devastated, particularly since my peers in the program treated me like a pariah because their workload increased. They showed me no compassion, which only added to my sense of loss and trauma.

I would look at myself in the mirror with disbelief. My body was whole! How could I be so drastically disabled? I now recognize those thoughts as internalized ableism. Ableism is the denial of disability, particularly when one does not *appear* disabled. It often leads to denial of employment, access to facilities and even sidewalks, inability to shop in stores, and limitations in health care and many other basic human needs. Internalized ableism is one's inability to accept disability. In my case, as I looked at my largely intact body, I found it extremely challenging to accept that I was disabled. I would continue trying to perform tasks that were beyond my physical limitations, and I would pay for it with unbearable pain. This furthered my emotional trauma and caused my denial to fester. When one can't see one's own injuries, it can be difficult, even additionally traumatizing, to accept them. It took many years to come to terms with my new reality, and at the time I felt deeply lost. People with hidden disabilities have created a sunflower symbol to display to others that we have hidden disabilities, but it is still extremely difficult to accept them for ourselves.

In my state I turned to the psalms. My training led me to Psalm 22, in which I found great comfort:

> My God, my God, why have you abandoned me?
> My God, I cry in the day, and You don't answer,
>   and at night I have no relief.
> I am a worm, not a human, scorned by people,
>   despised by humanity.
> Those who see me mock me. (Psalm 22:1, 22:3, 22:7–8)[1]

These verses capture the Psalmist's deep depression and trauma following a horrible experience. If you read the entire psalm, you would see that these verses are interspersed with more positive ones. But for me, in my intense emotional pain, the verses expressing the author's traumatic experience resonated with me the most. I felt that the Psalmist understood; they knew what it was like to survive trauma. I have always found power in Biblical texts, and having read a number of books on the healing power of psalms, I chose to turn to them in my pain. I had an index of psalms for specific needs, which led me to this psalm, and I remain very grateful for the guidance of those who brought me here.

During my disability journey, I read a book by Samuel Chiel and Henry Dreher titled *For Thou Art with Me: The Healing Power of Psalms*. This book did not include Psalm 22, but it showed how to derive power and growth from the psalms by pairing each psalm with a healing reflection. They write, for instance, of Psalm 68, "We communicate our burdens to God through the language of prayer."[2] This certainly proved true for me, as psalms became the way I most deeply communicated my pain and trauma to God.

Despite all the pain and trauma, I kept breathing and putting one foot in front of the other. This enabled me to reach a goal that was very important to me—completing rabbinical school. Before I retired from the military, I had a huge "aha" moment that I needed to pursue the rabbinic path rather than work as a defense contractor, which is what I was being groomed for. When I set my mind on a goal, I feel it is very important to achieve it. This goal actually existed in small pieces as a child, and had my childhood been different, I might have pursued the rabbinate much sooner. Still, rabbinical school was extremely challenging and a trauma in its own right, given how difficult the comprehensive examinations and courseload were. But I got through it. Very heavy pain pills kept my body together so I could do my work at the school, and I got it done.

I want to emphasize that despite the stigma around pain medication today, the medications I was taking were vital to my survival. In fact, today I live with severe *unmanaged* pain because of the current policies regarding pain medicines and management. I do not respond to the normative medications for the pain I suffer, so my options for treatment are pretty limited. This inability to properly manage my pain compounds my trauma, because I fully understand that this uncontrolled pain will shorten my life due to sleep deprivation, depression, cardiac disease, and many other ancillary conditions.

In addition to the joy of completing rabbinical school despite severe pain and disability, I also was finally able to discover my true self. It turned out that my pain medication interrupted the sex hormone stimulating hormone production. This caused a lot of physical and emotional issues in itself, but more significantly it led to a period of huge questioning and self-discovery. I wrote about this in my autobiography, *We Are God's Children Too*.[3] I had always been expressing my trans identity in different ways but didn't understand them. At this point in my life, I finally became open to understanding them and was able to discover my true self. I began my gender transition, becoming Rona. I've never been happier.

I have long applied the following metaphor to our interactions with the Divine. God presents us with a long hallway with a number of doorways. We can stand where we are, or we can move forward and choose a door, with its inherent risks and unknown rewards. This is where faith comes in and how God interacts with us. God gives us opportunities, but we need to be discerning and assertive to make the choice to walk through a particular door. I have walked through a lot of doors in my life, and I've never regretted one. But the one I'm most happy about is the one that gave me Rona. I've never been happier, even though I'm disabled, depressed, in pain, and traumatized.

I'm not saying that I'm happy about being disabled, depressed, in pain, and suffering trauma. Nobody would want any of that. I would much rather be healthy and working. But I don't suffer for lack of needs, as so many do. I have a wife, housing, food, health care, pets, and more—all of which offer support and help me cope. But my traumatic experiences have given me a deep understanding of suffering that enables me to be a compassionate listener, and I'm a great pastoral counselor because of it. In addition, my trauma led to my self-discovery, and I would never change that. For that reason, I say with complete faith:

אוֹדְךָ כִּי עֲנִיתָנִי וַתְּהִי־לִי לִישׁוּעָה:

I praise You, for You have answered me,
and You have been my Salvation! (Psalm 118:21)

NOTES

1. All psalm translations are by the author.
2. Samuel Chiel and Henry Dreher, *For Thou Art with Me: The Healing Power of Psalms* (Daybreak Books, 2000), 159.
3. Rabbah Rona Matlow, DMin, *We Are God's Children Too* (TransGender Publishing, 2020).

16

Radical Resistance

Overcoming Racial Trauma
to Build *Olam Chadash,* a New World

Yolanda Savage-Narva

I INVITE YOU to go on a journey with me for the next few pages—a journey that began in the womb of a young Black woman born in 1950 in Natchez, Mississippi, a city situated on the banks of the Mississippi River. In 1945, five years before she was born, World War II ended after the genocide of six million Jews. In 1955, five years after she was born, Emmett Till—a fourteen-year-old Black boy from Chicago—was murdered for whistling at a white woman in Money, Mississippi, igniting the civil rights movement. This child was born between two major world events, one framed by the Nuremberg Laws and the other by Jim Crow.[1] These were two distinct systems rooted in dehumanization, fear, death, and destruction based on socially constructed racial identities that continue to cause deep trauma for so many today.

By the time I was conceived twenty-two years later, my mother had moved north, which is where she met my father. He grew up in Chicago, Illinois, one of the northern cities along the Great Migration trail. Chicago was a haven for Black families as they moved north between 1916 and 1970 in search of better opportunities and to flee the horrors and injustices of the Jim Crow South. As it turns out, cities in the Midwest and Northeast offered only temporary respite and safety for families looking for a better life. Eventually, many Black families found themselves in segregated, overcrowded housing projects with the same atmosphere and intent as the European ghettos. They were designed to create separation and maintain "white purity." The result was a clear sense of otherness and despair.

The DNA passed on to me from my mother and father means that the experiences of their ancestors—the tragedies of genocides and enslavement—now live in me. My genes perpetuate trauma through my epigenetic journey.[2] This is a journey that I cannot change, but one that hopefully I can manage.

Navigating the world as a Black Jewish woman from the South, I find myself in continuous conversations with friends, family, colleagues, and strangers explaining, describing, and validating how each of my identities shapes who I am and how I exist in the world. At times these identities are in symmetry with one another, and at other times there is a dynamic tension that exists between them. In addition to these multiple identities, I am also a Jewish professional whose work is focused on creating vibrant equitable communities of belonging for all people. Because I navigate living with these multiple identities, it is critical that I have a way to manage the challenges that come with them.

An incident that stands out vividly in my mind happened several years ago when I led a nonprofit organization in Washington, DC. I sent an email solicitation out to supporters of the organization, informing them about a recent successful youth program. The email went out to the entire listserv. Many people enjoyed learning about the success of the program and decided to donate to the organization. But not everyone was happy with the program, or, as they called it, the "perceived program." A former board member decided to respond to the solicitation with racist, ugly accusations directed toward me. The email was addressed to "WTF" and included the accusation that I was exposing the students to antisemitic people, threats to never support the organization again, and degrading insults about my character and ability to lead. When I shared the email with the executive board and asked them to intervene, most of them were in total dismay and sickened by the email. One board member, however, wasn't convinced the accusations weren't true and questioned me about them. This pattern wasn't unusual for this board member. Throughout my tenure at this organization, he and several others consistently displayed racist and sexist behaviors and attitudes toward me. I couldn't believe what was happening. I felt demeaned and embarrassed by both incidents. I constantly felt like an imposter, second-guessing myself and wondering if I was worthy to be in my current role. Yes, I was hurt by the email, but the questioning by the board member—someone I had worked with for several years—wounded me in a way that was deep and everlasting.

When this happened, I had no idea how to cope with it or compartmentalize how the systemic nature of racism manifests itself in individual-to-individual encounters.

As I paired this story and so many others with the trauma I carry within my DNA, I realized I can offer some best and promising practices for how to navigate specific challenges. When I came to this realization, I knew I had to find something or someone bigger than myself—perhaps an ancient tradition—that I could rely on. As I searched for the answer, I asked myself the following four questions:

1. *WHAT DOES BEING JEWISH MEAN TO ME SPECIFICALLY?* Being Jewish means being whole; no part of who I am is wondering and searching for a place to belong. I am proud to be in the body I am in, and I embrace the complexity of who I am. Being Jewish allows me to tap into the diversity of how I navigate the world from a place of spiritual, religious, and cultural curiosity. To me, being Jewish also means having a sense of fulfillment. It allows me to be okay and satisfied with having more questions than answers, because our tradition welcomes the opportunity to wrestle and question. I do not feel conflicted or unfulfilled if all the questions haven't been answered. Being Jewish allows me to tap into a four-thousand-year-old tradition that is rooted in spirituality, curiosity, and empathy. Our tradition believes that every living and breathing thing has a heart, has a purpose, can feel pain and joy, and carries a spark of divinity.

2. *HOW DOES MY UNIQUE PRACTICE OF JUDAISM GIVE ME THE TOOLS TO NAVIGATE THE WORLD?* In 2021, I was invited to join a cohort of like-minded individuals to learn and be trained in Mussar and Kabbalah. I was looking for the strength and stamina to continue the work of creating vibrant and equitable communities of belonging. Unlike many people, I did not log off my computer and put my work aside. My work is intimately connected with who I am and how I live my life, day in and day out. My toolbox is filled with both religious and spiritual practices. Mussar and Kabbalah practices focus on healing the world from the inside out. I find myself connecting closely with several Mussar practices that ground me in sacred text while providing me with opportunities for diversity of expression. *Hitpaalut, hitbod'dut, cheshbon hanefesh*, and *chavruta*, are my "go-to" practices.

Hitpaalut/hispailus (focus phrase) is commonly understood as ecstatic prayer when one phrase is repeated. As I learned in my training, *hitpaalut/hispailus* is an anchoring focus phrase connected to a *midah* (character trait). For example, I anchor myself in a *midah* such as *kavod* (dignity) and chant the phrase "You have to learn to leave the table when love is no longer being served."[3] This phrase and many others have helped me in situations where people are disrespectful toward me and my work. Research has shown a strong correlation between trauma and the pathology-inducing responses frequently experienced by Black women.

Hitbod'dut (solitude) is understood as "intimately talking to God," and it allows me to feel the presence of *HaShem* (God) everywhere. I prefer to be outdoors when I am engaged in *hitbod'dut*, but I can have conversations with God anywhere. I find that doing this practice every day can be immensely powerful. I do not wait to have conversations with God until there is a crisis or something urgent. Rather, I enjoy the frequency of conversations with God that feel more like I am building a meaningful relationship.

Cheshbon hanefesh (accounting of the soul) can be done anytime. For me, *cheshbon hanefesh* is best done through journaling. On a train, in between meetings, at night before I go to bed, or in the morning when I first wake up. My journaling is usually connected to another practice such as listening to a *nigun* (wordless melody) or after a meditation or *hitbod'dut*.

Chavruta (friendship, companionship) is usually small-group or partnered text study and can be done online or in person. *Chavruta* has informally and formally been a big part of my spiritual journey for many years. A couple of years ago, I set up weekly *chavruta* sessions with rabbis and cantors. It was such a fulfilling experience, and I plan to repeat it in the future.

3. *WHAT IS UNIQUE ABOUT MY PROXIMITY TO TRAUMA?* Black and Jewish trauma overlap in many regards, though each community has its unique experiences with trauma and pain throughout history. The more recent enslavement of people of African descent and the Biblical enslavement of the Hebrews in Egypt are two very well-known tragic examples. Both

communities have also been traumatized by other systemic forms of terror. One example is pogroms—violent riots that intend to destroy an ethnic, racial, or religious group. In 1903, a pogrom in Kishinev (present-day Moldova) killed dozens of Jews. In 1921, the Tulsa Massacre killed hundreds of Black Americans. In the United States, experiences with discrimination and segregation continued to plague both Black Americans and Jews well into the 1960s (specifically in the South). Of course, racism and antisemitism continue to be present today in various degrees and iterations. More recent incidents—the deadly attack on innocent congregants at Pittsburgh's Tree of Life Synagogue in 2018, the white supremacist rally in Charlottesville in 2019, the brutal murder of George Floyd in 2020, the Buffalo grocery store mass shooting in 2022—are directly connected to the underlying systemic oppression that people from all marginalized backgrounds face in this country. It is also particularly important to note that these two communities are not binary. There are people like me who are both Black and Jewish. Although only one of those identities is obvious, both are very much a part of who I am today and how I navigate the world. At times, especially after the horrific attack by Hamas in Israel on October 7, 2023, the intersections of these two identities have become even more complex to navigate, both within the Jewish community and in the broader community. I have often felt like I was in the middle of a tug-of-war—being pulled in two different directions at once—and at the same time feeling almost invisible and ignored. There are assumptions made—primarily from the Jewish community, but from the Black community as well— that I can't possibly have anything to say about what's happening in Israel/Palestine, because I don't "fit" the way people think about the Black experience in this country and I don't "fit" the way people think about the Jewish experience in this country. We often experience both racism and antisemitism together in the same orbit, and at times we experience racism in one orbit and antisemitism in another. Although many of the most horrific events our communities have experienced happened a long time ago, the scars, the fear, the trauma, and the unresolved emotions never actually go away. We must begin to understand and acknowledge how trauma impacts our everyday lives.

4. WHAT IS MY CALL TO ACTION FOR OLAM CHADASH *(creating a new world)?* To create a new world, the cycle of trauma must be broken. I recognize that I do not have the ability to rewire DNA. I cannot go back to the past and rewrite history. I cannot erase the enslavement of Africans and their descendants, erase the Holocaust, or erase any other racial, ethnic, or national trauma. And while the horrific events of the past continue to haunt us, we are also currently responsible for the pain and suffering happening to so many in the world around us.

In the new world that I dream of, day one would be a day of the living. No one would be allowed to intentionally take a life. There would be no gun violence on the streets, no shooting missiles, and no torture. In the new world that I dream of, this single act of valuing every life would recalibrate the imbalance in the universe and send vibrations of hope, love, compassion, resiliency, and joy into the atmosphere. These would be felt in the hearts, souls, spirits, and minds of every living being on this planet. As Dr. Martin Luther King Jr. said, "True peace is not merely the absence of tension; it is the presence of justice."[4] For true healing, we must resist the urge to do what people do when they experience trauma—retreat to their corners, lose their sense of empathy for others, and focus only on their specific pain. I don't have the luxury of retreating to one corner over the other. I cannot retreat to the "Black people's corner" or the "Jewish people's corner," because I share both identities. I am relying on my intersecting identities as my superpower to bring Black people who aren't Jewish and Jewish people who aren't Black closer together to realize the sacred humanity in one another and to allow us—even at this very challenging time in history—to see each other through the lens of *b'tzelem Elohim* (the image of God). It is very painful and heartbreaking to watch the moral arc of the universe bending away from justice, solidarity, and liberation for all people. If we don't have the tools to navigate terrible events in our lives or our world, our response is one rooted in a trauma response. Instead, we must recognize that our safety, sanity, sacredness, and shared humanity are connected to our solidarity. We are *all* the keepers of the land, keepers of the people, and keepers of the covenant.

NOTES

1. The Nazis closely studied American race laws and the ways that Jim Crow policies discriminated against Black Americans. See Becky Little, "How the Nazis Were Inspired by Jim Crow," HISTORY, August 4, 2023, https://www.history.com/news/how-the-nazis-were-inspired-by-jim-crow.

2. "Epigenetics (also sometimes called epigenomics) is a field of study focused on changes in DNA that do not involve alterations to the underlying sequence. The DNA letters and the proteins that interact with DNA can have chemical modifications that change the degrees to which genes are turned on and off. Certain epigenetic modifications may be passed on from parent cell to daughter cell during cell division or from one generation to the next." See "Epigenetics," Genome.gov, n.d., https://www.genome.gov/genetics-glossary/Epigenetics. See also Rachel Yehuda, "How Parents' Trauma Leaves Biological Traces in Children," *Scientific American*, February 20, 2024, https://www.scientificamerican.com/article/how-parents-rsquo-trauma-leaves-biological-traces-in-children/; and Aziz Elbasheir et al., "Racial Discrimination, Neural Connectivity, and Epigenetic Aging Among Black Women," *JAMA Network Open* 7, no. 6 (June 13, 2024): e2416588, https://doi.org/10.1001/jamanetworkopen.2024.16588.

3. Nina Simone, vocalist, "You've Got to Learn," by Charles Aznavour and Marcel Stellman, track 11 on *I Put a Spell on You*, Philips Records, 1965.

4. Martin Luther King Jr., *Stride Toward Freedom: The Montgomery Story* (Harper & Row, 1958).

PART FOUR

Trauma from Personal and Communal Violence

17

Esther, Sexual Assault, and the Winding Road of Healing

Rabbi Iah Pillsbury

In the middle of the night, in the dark and shadows, the pain and hurt feel closer, though still far away. It didn't used to feel like this. There used to be no distance, no breath between the memory of violation and the feeling of it in the here and now. Healing didn't seem possible. At times, neither did survival. And then somehow, between all the therapy and the painting and the journaling, the talking and the silence and the changing everything about how I lived and structured my life, everything about how I saw myself and related to others, something shifted profoundly. Here I am, the pain somehow a distant memory rather than my daily, all-consuming reality.

I didn't always know what happened to me. Some of it I knew, but not all. I struggled with labeling what happened, even the stuff I did know about and that happened when I was a young adult. It just felt bad and wrong. It was confusing. She was my best friend. I had liked her. We had been together many times before. And yet, that time was different. Violation is complicated like that. Rape isn't always obvious and dramatic, the way it is portrayed in so many movies. Often it is ambiguous and hidden. It can be hard to see and even harder to name.

I have always been a feminist. I always firmly believed that no one is ever "asking for it" and that the victim or survivor is never at fault. And yet, when it was me—especially the child me—somehow it didn't feel that way. I felt dirty and ashamed. I felt like my victimhood was a beacon that everyone could see. I felt like I was somehow complicit. I felt like what happened to me as a child and as a young adult somehow made me "less than," less worthy of the good things in life, and less worthy of trust and respect. I was too broken. Too scared. I somehow believed that the brokenness and fear were my fault and that I was both tainted and contagious. If anyone got too close to me or listened, I worried it would rub off on them and hurt them. So I tucked myself away and hid from those I wasn't already close to. Everything and everyone was a possible threat. Every touch. Every glance. Every time I left my house. Every time I went to sleep.

I remember sitting in one of many support groups for survivors, looking around the room at the other participants and being astounded— thinking, *they* don't look like something like this happened to them. They don't look like they would *let* anyone treat them that way. They look too strong for that. Or too put together. Or too untouchable. I wondered if I would ever be in that place myself. I desperately wanted to be.

And then I met Esther. I had, of course, always known the story of Esther. When I was a child, Purim was always one of my favorite holidays. What could be better than a silly, costumed holiday featuring two awesome women, one who defied the king and the other who saved our people from the evil Haman's plot to kill the Jews? Then one day, one of my professors at rabbinical school asked, "Well, you do know Esther was a rape victim, right?" And I just stopped. I was floored. ESTHER?? The powerful, larger-than-life Esther who saved our people? Why had no one ever told me? I couldn't believe it and yet I felt the truth of it deep inside me like a breath releasing.

As we discussed Esther and I thought about the Biblical story more deeply, my professor's comment made more and more sense. Her victimization and violation were hiding right in plain sight, just like so many people's real-life stories and experiences. In the Biblical narrative, we first meet Esther as a beautiful orphan, raised by her older cousin Mordecai.[1] She is vulnerable from the very beginning, not only as a young woman, but as a young woman without parents. As soon as we meet Esther, she and other young virgins are taken to the palace for the king, Ahasuerus, to choose from. They spend a year in captivity in the harem being groomed for the king's pleasure, and then they are taken night after night for the king to "try out." According to the Biblical text itself, when Esther is brought to him, the king loves her, and she becomes queen.[2] When I was growing up, this story was told as if the girls were competing in a beauty pageant. We were told that it was a huge success that the Jewish girl Esther was considered the most beautiful and became the queen of Persia. There was no acknowledgment of what we would, in modern terms, call sex trafficking and sexual slavery. There was no acknowledgment or discussion of the lack of consent, of the fear these girls must have felt, of the age difference between them and the king, of what captivity and the nights with the king must have cost them.

The Rabbinic literature about Esther tells an even darker, more painful story. It is a story of incest and repeated violations, of dissociation and the losing of self, of being trapped and yet finding strength and agency amid the harm.

The Babylonian Talmud, *M'gillah* 12a–15b functions as an extended midrashic text, telling stories about the Biblical tale of Esther that both support and compete with each other. When we meet Esther in *M'gillah* 13a, Mordecai not only adopts her as a baby, but also takes her for a wife in back-to-back teachings.[3] So it is as a victim of incest that Esther comes to the palace to once again be used by men in power, first potentially by Hegai—the keeper of women (see Esther 2:8–9)—and then by King Ahasuerus. *M'gillah* 13a teaches that even Esther's most secret and private part of herself, her sexuality and virginity,[4] is not her own, but dependent on the desire of the king. It is that dependence that ends up winning her the crown. Once Esther becomes queen, she is still caught between Mordecai and the king, still struggling to find agency over herself and her body—"She maintained a relationship with Mordecai, as she would arise from the lap of Ahasuerus, immerse herself in a ritual bath [mikveh], and sit in the lap of Mordecai" (*M'gillah* 13b). Here "sitting in the lap" of Mordecai and the king is a euphemism for being used sexually by both men (hence the need for the immersion in the mikveh to purify herself between encounters), since it is understood by the Rabbis that she could not consent to either relationship.[5]

And yet, even with all the victimization and exploitation that Esther survives, she still emerges as a powerful woman with agency and as one of the seven prophetesses of Israel.[6] She does the impossible when no one else can or will, risking everything to save her people. She is not weak in our version of her story, but incredibly, indescribably strong. In the end, when it really matters, she tells Mordecai what to do. Then after fasting and reflection, she wraps herself in royalty (*malchut*),[7] or, as the

Rabbis understand it, the Divine Presence (*Shechinah*),[8] and approaches the king of her own volition. Despite all that Esther has been through, according to *M'gillah* 15b,[9] the Divine Presence leaves her, and in the end, she is all alone, crying out, "My God, my God, why have You forsaken me?" (Psalm 22:2). Though God is not mentioned in the Biblical Book of Esther, the Rabbis of the Talmud imagine Esther holding God accountable to some extent, unafraid to voice her feelings of betrayal and anger. Yet, even then, she continues and approaches the king, an act that the Rabbis understand to mean that she gives herself to him sexually. She sacrifices herself to save her people. And at that moment, Esther becomes *karka olam*, the "dirt of the earth" or "natural ground."[10] For the Rabbis, this meant that Esther was not liable for approaching the king sexually—she wasn't an active participant. It was happening to her, like the earth that has no say in where or how the farmer plows.

Karka olam—the natural ground. I have never come across a more perfect description of what it means to dissociate, to not really be there in your body when terrible things are happening to it. There is a hollowness, a surreality, and also a hyperreality. There is passivity, but the act of dissociation can also be understood as an act of agency and rebellion. It means that as much as someone tries to violate you, they can't really touch you because you're not *really* there. Of course, just like so many coping mechanisms that are helpful in the moment, dissociation can continue to occur and become much less helpful and more painful. It can be incredibly frightening and make us feel out of control. It can come upon us seemingly out of nowhere and become a cycle that is difficult to break or change. And yet, when we can embrace it and ask ourselves why dissociation is here with more curiosity than judgment, things may begin to shift. We begin to learn more about ourselves and our stories, about our needs and what is and isn't working for us—about what we may need to change in our lives, both internally and externally.

My journey of healing, like all journeys, has not been linear or straightforward. It has moved in spirals and circles, doubling back and moving forward. Sometimes it has felt insurmountable, and other times healing happened when I wasn't paying attention. One breath, one nightmare, one moment of beauty, one boundary set and upheld at a time. And it is a journey, I know, that will never end but will continue to unfold and change during the entirety of my life. Throughout my journey, I have been grateful to have found friends and mentors, mental health professionals and spiritual leaders, texts and teachings and traditions that have bolstered me and helped to create the many paths of healing I have benefited from.

During rabbinical school, before I met Esther in the fullness of her story, I spent a year living with my then eighty-five-year-old grandfather and going to therapy. I think of that year as my year of healing, even though my healing work began before then and continued long after. I went to therapy four times a week, took part in a support group and bodywork[11] weekly, and spent time with my awesome grandfather and his fabulous friends. They were all New York Reform Jews who liked to complain about religion and temple and yet would never dream of not being full dues-paying members. All had served in World War II or had spouses who served. All had seen terrible things and then had come home and built a new and beautiful life in the shadows of trauma. All loved to talk about how the magical nature of religion and God did not make sense, especially when there was so much suffering in the world, and yet every year, they all said *Kaddish* for their spouses, children, and parents on the anniversaries of their deaths. They were a breath of fresh air for me and gave me the space I needed to continue my own journey of belief (or lack thereof) in God and our tradition. I spent time asking myself what it all meant and what the point was, eventually beginning to find and articulate meaning again.

My grandfather was in his early twenties at the end of the war and spent time near the concentration camps after they had been liberated, digging graves and helping folks who were still there get home or find a new home. He was haunted by those memories, by this time in his life when he witnessed the effects of evil and felt like he couldn't do anything about it—a time that never made sense, no matter how often he thought about it or talked about it. I, too, was dealing with a time in my life that didn't make sense, a time when people had done terrible things that I had suppressed. We ate together and laughed together, talked together, and played with the cat together while we wrestled with the terrible deeds humans can do to one another.

When I wasn't hanging out with my grandfather or with my new support-group friends or in therapy, I was painting. Specifically, I painted Psalm 22, the same psalm the Rabbis believe Esther cried out before approaching the king—though when I started I did not know this connection to Esther; I just felt abandoned and confused. *"My God, my God, why have You forsaken me?"* I painted line after line of the psalm, letting the horrors I had experienced pour out of me in vivid watercolors, giving each line new meaning and often adding bits of Hebrew to the text itself. It felt important to illustrate what I had trouble speaking and to integrate our tradition with my own story. It was meaningful to use my ancestor's words to struggle with God again, to give voice to my pain and heartache, the feelings of hurt and betrayal. It helped me feel less alone, and it also helped me release some of the pain of my own story. It helped me to move it outside of myself, so I could look at it when I needed to, but not obsess about it constantly.

My journey of healing has been full of many kinds of therapy and art: journaling, painting, dance, music, energy work, EMDR, brainspotting,[12] and leaning on loved ones. I have spent a lot of time reading, writing, talking, and being. It used to hurt to let myself feel the good stuff in life; I could barely tolerate it. And so I learned to sit and pet my cat, feel her purr, and try to just be present in the moment. I tried to take in the safety and the beauty, to breathe it into myself and focus on how it felt in tiny fragments and then in larger and larger pieces. I learned to cry again and to embrace myself more deeply. I began to remind myself of my own worthiness and the many possibilities that lived on the other side of survival. Somehow, despite my biggest fears, it worked. Things are fundamentally different now.

Esther's story is a story of a survivor. She is someone who experienced true terror and yet lived through it. It is a story we are commanded to hear every year. Even if we don't often hear the complete version, the commandment is still there. It is a powerful reminder that hearing our stories and giving voice to our pain is important. It doesn't diminish us. Surviving terrible hurt and violation does not make us less than or greater than; it just makes us, us. Esther's story reminds us that true strength can be hiding in plain sight and that if and when we are ready, our stories deserve to be told.

NOTES

1. All Biblical translations are from *The JPS Tanakh: Gender-Sensitive Edition* (Jewish Publication Society, 2023), found on Sefaria (sefaria.org). Esther 2:7: "He was foster father to Hadassah—that is, Esther—his uncle's daughter, for she had neither father nor mother. The maiden was shapely and beautiful; and when her father and mother died, Mordecai adopted her as his own daughter."

2. Esther 2:17: "The king loved Esther more than all the other women, and she won his grace and favor more than all the virgins. So he set a royal diadem on her head and made her queen instead of Vashti."

3. Translations of the Babylonian Talmud are from the William Davidson digital edition of the *Koren Noé Talmud*, with commentary by Rabbi Adin Even-Israel Steinsaltz (license: CC-BY-NC, https://creativecommons. org/licenses/by-nc/4.0/), found on Sefaria. The bold text of the quotation is a direct translation. The text in plain type was added in English in order to create full sentences (and explain what the Talmud assumes the reader already knows). Babylonian Talmud, *M'gillah* 13a: "The verse initially states with regard to Esther: '**For she had neither father nor mother'** (Esther 2:7). **Why do I need** to be told in the continuation of the verse: '**And when her father and mother were dead,** Mordecai took her for his own daughter'? **Rav Aḥa said:** This repetition indicates that **when** her mother **became pregnant** with her, **her father died,** and **when she gave birth** to her, **her mother died,** so that she did not have a mother or a father for even a single day. The verse states: '**And when her father and mother were dead, Mordecai took her for his own daughter'** (Esther 2:7). A *tanna* [a scholar from the first and second centuries CE] **taught** a *baraita* [a Rabbinic teaching by a *tanna* that was not included in the Mishnah] **in the name of Rabbi Meir: Do not read** the verse literally as **for a daughter [*bat*],** but **rather** read it as **for a home [*bayit*].** This indicates that Mordecai took Esther to be his wife. **And so it states: 'But the poor man had nothing, except one little ewe lamb, which he had bought and reared: And it grew up together with him, and with his children; it did eat of his bread, and drank of his own cup, and lay in his bosom, and was like a daughter [*kevat*] to him'** (II Samuel 12:3). The Gemara questions: **Because it lay in his bosom, it 'was like a daughter to him'? Rather,** the parable in II Samuel referenced the illicit taking of another's wife, and the phrase should be read: **Like a home [*bayit*] to him,** i.e., a wife. **So too, here,** Mordecai took her **for a home,** i.e., a wife."

4. Babylonian Talmud, *M'gillah* 13a: "**If** [the king] **wanted to taste** in her **the taste of a virgin** during intercourse, **he tasted it,** and if he wanted to experience **the taste of a non-virgin, he tasted it.**"

5. According to the *Tosafot* commenting on *K'tubot* 26b, it can be assumed that a captive woman would try to seduce her prison guards in order to potentially win her freedom. This means that a woman who is in captivity is not capable of consent, since it is expected that she will do anything she can to survive, including any act that appears sexual to the observer.

6. Babylonian Talmud, *M'gillah* 14a: "The Gemara [Rabbinic commentary on the Mishnah] asks with regard to the prophetesses recorded in the *baraita*: **Who were the seven prophetesses?** The Gemara answers: **Sarah, Miriam, Deborah, Hannah, Abigail, Huldah, and Esther.**"

7. Esther 5:1: "On the third day, Esther put on royal apparel and stood in the inner court of the king's palace, facing the king's palace, while the king was sitting on his royal throne in the throne room facing the entrance of the palace."

8. Babylonian Talmud, *M'gillah* 14b: "**Esther** was also a prophetess, **as it is written: 'And it came to pass on the third day that Esther clothed herself in royalty'** (Esther 5:1). **It should have said:** Esther clothed herself in **royal garments. Rather,** this alludes to the fact **that she clothed herself with a divine** spirit of **inspiration. It is written here: 'And she clothed herself,' and it is written elsewhere: 'And the spirit clothed Amasai'** (I Chronicles 12:19)."

9. Babylonian Talmud, *M'gillah* 15b: "**Rabbi Levi said: Once she reached the chamber of the idols,** which was in the inner court, **the Divine Presence left her. She** immediately **said: 'My God, my God, why have You forsaken me?'** (Psalms 22:2). **Perhaps** it is because **You judge an unintentional sin as one** performed **intentionally, and** an action **done due to** circumstances **beyond one's control as** one done **willingly.**"

10. Babylonian Talmud, *Sanhedrin* 74b: "**But wasn't** the incident involving **Esther,** i.e., her cohabitation with Ahasuerus, **a public** sin? Why then did Esther not surrender her life rather than engage in intercourse? The Gemara answers: **Abaye says: Esther was** merely like **natural ground,** i.e., she was a passive participant. The obligation to surrender one's life rather than engage in forbidden sexual intercourse applies only to a man who transgresses the prohibition in an active manner. A woman who is passive and merely submits is not required to give up her life so that she not sin."

11. Bodywork is a kind of therapy that helps release trauma and hurts that are held in the physical body. It uses touch, massage, the sacral-facial system, various pressure points, and movement.

12. All of these therapeutic techniques are different ways of releasing trauma and helping to process it in layers. EMDR (eye movement desensitiza-

tion and reprocessing) uses bilateral stimulation to rewire neural pathways. Brainspotting uses eye positioning to access the subcortical brain. See emdria.org and brainspotting.com for more information.

18

From the Narrow Places

The Trauma of Gun Violence

RABBI JOEL MOSBACHER

IN HIS REMARKABLE VOLUME *The Body Keeps the Score*, Dr. Bessel van der Kolk writes, "The past is alive in the form of gnawing interior discomfort."[1]

When I think about the call I got on January 19, 1999, at 9:43 a.m., just six months after I was ordained as a rabbi, I viscerally feel Dr. van der Kolk's words. I can still see the clock on my office wall in my mind's eye and hear my aunt's sobbing voice on the other end of the line: "Your father was shot; I think you should come now."

The shock I felt at that moment turned to panic as I ran through the Atlanta airport to catch a plane to Chicago. Within hours, it turned to grief as I recited *Vidui*, the confessional prayer, on my father's behalf. These feelings still sit with me twenty-five years later. There was no time for goodbye; another human being, created in the image of the Divine, chose to murder my father with a gun.

I had never recited *Vidui* before, but the words of the prayer that my rabbi, Leo Wolkow, *z"l*, read to me over the phone, so that I could recite them for my father, grounded me in the most ungrounded moment of my life. They allowed me to verbalize what I knew to be true: My father was a good man who had always done the best he could in life, despite how brutally his life was stolen from him and, by extension, from my family and me.

Even now, as I write these words, a part of me is still in denial that this is how my beloved father died.

I have worked as an organizer committed to reducing the scourge of gun violence for more than a decade. I know from so many personal stories that no American is more than a few degrees removed from this plague. While not every American has firsthand experience, we all are touched by this trauma. We are so accustomed to the frequency of death by gun in America that it is easy to be numbed by it. But I will never be numb.

I found myself caught between my own needs and the needs of my congregants, as perhaps clergy do in many circumstances. I had my own experience of this tragedy, and I needed (and continue to need) to process it in my own way, grieve and rail against the universe, crawl into a hole sometimes, punch a wall (just once), and get a whole lot of therapy. In *Pirkei Avot* 1:14, Rabbi Hillel asks, "If I am not for myself, who will be for me?" I understood that I had to take care of myself and express my authentic feelings. No one would do that for me, and I would be no good for others if I wasn't present for what was true in my own soul. I made the time to be with my wife and my friends, to visit my mom often, to start therapy, and most of all, to roll around on the floor with my one-year-old.

At the same time, as a rabbi, I was and am often invited to be present with others in their trauma. And while, thankfully, I haven't experienced every kind of trauma, and even though I'd give back what my family and I went through to be a little less effective as a pastor but have my dad back, I admit that having gone through the narrow places of my own experience, I can perhaps more effectively tap into that experience to be present for others. Hillel continues, "If I am only for myself, what am I?" I knew that I still wanted to live a life that was also a part of being present with others in their joys and in their sorrows. Even though it felt hard to be fully present for the goodness and pain in other people's lives in the first weeks and months after my father's death, those sacred moments, in many ways, brought me back to life. Through sharing the joys and pains of others, I gradually came to find that I could rejoice again and that I could also be present for the sadness of others. I could still be a person of faith; I could still be a rabbi.

During rabbinical school at Hebrew Union College–Jewish Institute of Religion in Cincinnati, our teacher Rabbi Julie Schwartz assured our clinical pastoral education group that we would be fine pastors, even if we hadn't had cancer, gone through a divorce, suffered the death of a child, been fired, or a thousand other things that our congregants would have experienced. "Do you know what loss feels like? What grief feels like? What pain feels like? If so, you can be present to the pain and grief and loss of others." That is Torah that I lean on nearly every day of my rabbinate.

In an essay on *Parashat Chayei Sarah* in *The Mussar Torah Commentary*, Rabbi Jennifer Gubitz teaches us about the trauma that Isaac went through as a result of the *Akeidah* (the Binding of Isaac) followed immediately by the death of his mother. Rabbi Gubitz asks why Isaac's voice was suddenly silent:

> Some commentators actually suggest this silence was a permanent and final departure—that the trauma was so painful that he died of fear. Others imagine he was blinded. Other commentaries envision that it was neither death nor illness, but rather that Isaac's departure was a multifaceted journey of resilience and recovery. *B'reishit Rabbah* teaches that after the *Akeidah*, Isaac went to study in a *beit midrash*, a "house of learning." Drowning his sorrows and his past in the books and traditions of our people, he immersed in a community of learners and seekers.[2]

In so many ways, after my father was murdered, I did what *B'reishit Rabbah* advised. I immersed myself more deeply in my family and my community. As I felt like I was drowning in grief and anger, I found a life preserver in words of Torah.

From a place of despair, sitting through an appeals trial that would acquit a man who had earlier been convicted of the murder, I thought often of the words of the Psalmist. I read Psalm 44 repeatedly. On the one hand, the Psalmist writes, "O God, through our ears we have heard, our ancestors told us stories: a work You worked in their days, in days of old" (verse 2). On the other hand, they write, "Why have You hidden Your face? You have forgotten our affliction, our oppression" (verse 25).

As I lost hope of understanding why a man would do this to my dear father, I clung desperately to the words of Psalm 118:5, "From within the narrow space I cried out: Yah! The Holy One answered me in Yah's expansive space." Even in the depths of my sorrow, I knew that I was seeking answers to unanswerable questions. With time—gradually, slowly, unevenly—I came to find that while I might never know why, I could find relief and comfort in our tradition, in the people around me, and in God's presence in my life.

When Yom Kippur came around in the year 2000, I heard the words of Deuteronomy 30:19 with new ears, new appreciation, and new resolve. "I have put before you life and death, blessing and curse. Choose life—if you and your offspring would live." I knew that for my own sake, for my wife and child, for my mom, and, yes, for my dad, I wanted to choose to continue to live my life to its fullest, to continue to see the goodness and possibility in the world, even if the gnawing interior discomfort that van der Kolk speaks of would never disappear.

And in those first months after his death, I read the words of the Mourner's *Kaddish* as if for the first time. I always knew that the prayer didn't speak of death, but when I read it after my father was killed, I came to realize that, for me, it was a kind of fake-it-till-you-make-it prayer. It asserts that there is goodness in the universe, even when we can't find the words to speak; it implores us to pray for abundant peace and life for us all, even as we might be in the depths of our deepest sorrow and doubt. Though we may be struck mute by loss, *Kaddish* calls mourners to pray words of hope and affirmation until, perhaps, we come to believe those words and prayers again.

Nothing can undo the trauma of my father's death; nothing can bring him back to my mother, my family, or me. There will always be a sadness in my soul as I mourn his untimely and wholly unnecessary death. But I know what pain and loss feel like. I know what it is like to walk through the narrowest places, to walk through the dark night of the soul, and what it's like to come out on the other side, wounded but whole. I know that my father would want me to live, to laugh, to remember better days, and to give whatever wholeness I have to my family, to my people, and to the world. With the blessing of his memory and with the strength of the Holy One of Blessing, it's what I try, imperfectly, to do each and every day.

NOTES
1. Bessel A. van der Kolk, *The Body Keeps the Score* (Penguin Books, 2015), 97.
2. Jennifer A. Gubitz, "*Chayei Sarah: M'nuchat HaNefesh*," in *The Mussar Torah Commentary: A Spiritual Path to Living a Meaningful and Ethical Life*, ed. Barry H. Block (CCAR Press, 2020), 31–32.

19

Running into the Flames

A Jewish, Army National Guard and Army Reserve Response to Trauma

RABBI AARON A. STUCKER-ROZOVSKY

The opinions herein are those of the author and do not reflect the positions, policies, or opinions of the United States Army or the Department of Defense. The author is solely responsible for his work and not the content or opinions of the other authors, contributors, and editors of the rest of this publication.

IMAGINE your child's high school math or history teacher or middle school football coach, your local mechanic, or your CPA. They're going through their lesson plan, guiding a practice, changing the oil in your car, or filing your taxes. All of a sudden, they get a call. They literally, and I do mean literally, stop what they're doing, change into their camouflage uniforms, grab their go-bags, and drive to their armory or reserve center. They have no idea where they're going, when they'll be back, and in some cases, if they'll even make it back. These are not full-time soldiers at a distant Army base you've never heard of; they are your friends and neighbors, and they put it all on the line because they believe in you and something greater than themselves.

This is the story of the Army National Guard and Army Reserve.

When I think of the word "trauma," my first thought is always "Who's coming to the rescue, who's going to run into the flames?" In other words, I've always believed that the fires of trauma are best quenched by the waters of selfless service. When our ancestors were enslaved in Egypt, God sent Moses and Aaron to Pharaoh's court with the demand, "Let My people go" (Exodus 9:1). In the Holocaust, it was the paratroopers of the 101st "Screaming Eagles" Airborne Division, tankers of the 10th Armored Division, and "grunts" (foot soldiers) of the 4th, 45th, and 42nd Infantry Divisions who liberated Dachau.[1] On 9/11, it was the firefighters of the FDNY and cops of the NYPD who raced up the twin towers to rescue as many people as they could. Their reaction to trauma was the highest reassurance to others and a north star in my life.

There have been two verses of *chochmah* (wisdom) from our ancestors that have guided me throughout my life. The first is the declaration of the prophet Isaiah to *HaShem*, "Here I am. Send me!" (Isaiah 6:8). The second is from the sage Ben Azzai, who teaches in the seminal ethical work *Pirkei Avot* (Ethics of Our Fathers), "Run to do even a slight mitzvah" (4:2).[2] I've tried my best to live up to these holy words. Both of these teachings influenced my decisions not only to become a rabbi but also to enlist in the Army National Guard and Army Reserve.

From the colonial era and the War of Independence to the Civil War to the World Wars through 9/11 and today, National Guard and reserve forces have actually been some of the first military forces to respond in times of crisis and war.[3] Furthermore, for much of our nation's history, these part-time warriors constituted the bulk of America's combat power.[4]

But it's not just war. Whether it's responding to a natural disaster (Hurricanes Sandy and Katrina, tornadoes in the heartland, and forest fires out West), to riots and civil disturbances, or to the COVID pandemic, by setting up field hospitals, running tests, and respectfully transporting the remains of those who died, Army National Guards and Army Reserve soldiers have been at the forefront of keeping their communities safe both at home and abroad.[5]

Since 9/11, the Army National Guard and Army Reserve are no longer the "weekend warriors" that stereotyped previous generations of the force. They are battle-hardened and experienced formations who have years of consistent back-to-back deployments to the far reaches of the globe. In many instances, such as my own Army National Guard 2011–12 deployment to Afghanistan, reserve component units have even commanded active-duty forces.[6] This is without even discussing the multitude of domestic missions these forces have tackled. During the Cold War, the Army National Guard and Army Reserve were seen and often saw themselves as a "strategic reserve"—the nation's last line of defense.[7] Today, however, the reserve components are an integral and invaluable part of the national defense strategy.[8] To put it bluntly, the old adage of "one weekend a month, two weeks in the summer" is dead. There is no going back to the old days; there are simply too many threats in our world.

Essentially, I think the Army National Guards and Army Reserve soldiers live in two worlds. In Isaiah we are given the aspirational message "They shall beat their swords into plowshares and their spears into pruning hooks: Nation shall not take up sword against nation; they shall never again know war" (Isaiah 2:4). On the one hand, they are the farmer holding the plowshare and the pruning hook, and on the other hand, they are the soldier holding the sword and spear. They are realists who want to live in a world of peace, but like the minutemen of Lexington and Concord, they are ready to exchange the plow for the musket at a moment's notice in order to defend that which they love and hold dear.

When one's calling and duty is to run into the flames—by responding to Ground Zero after 9/11, sifting through the rubble looking for survivors or victims after a tornado in Kentucky or after Hurricane Katrina in New Orleans, or mounting daily patrols along the same stretch of contested road in Iraq or Afghanistan that had claimed the lives and limbs of friends only days before—there is no way that the Army Guards or Army Reserve soldiers will not be affected by what they have witnessed and experienced. Active-duty units may redeploy to a major installation where they are surrounded by fellow soldiers, but when Army National Guards and Army Reserve soldiers come home and are released from active duty, they return to their towns and cities, surrounded by civilian friends and neighbors. In addition, during World War II and the draft era (1940–73), service members and veterans were a far more common sight; today, these populations are a small minority (6 percent are veterans, and less than 1 percent serve on active duty).[9] This is not to say the American public is hostile or uncaring to our service members and veterans (far from it, in fact). Still, how can someone who has never been in a gunfight or combat understand that sense of adrenaline and fear that comes with seeing stacked garbage bags on the side of the highway, or even the constant need to switch up the route by which they go to work? All of these can potentially cause trauma and induce traumatic

responses in veterans and service members. Fortunately, the Department of Defense recognized this, and there are many avenues to help
service members and veterans of all components (active duty, Army
National Guard, and Army Reserve) as well as their families deal with
their experiences. These include (but are not limited to) support from
the VA, behavioral health and chaplain support, Yellow Ribbon events,
and various armed forces programs like Military OneSource, Master
Resilience Training, Combat and Operational Stress Control, and
Building Strong and Resilient Teams.[10] One of the best things an Army
National Guard or Army Reserve unit can do after demobilization is to
stay in touch, hang out, and ultimately talk, laugh, cry, and remember
what were some of the best and toughest days of their lives. Why? In
Henry V, Shakespeare writes, "And gentlemen in England now a-bed /
Shall think themselves accursed they were not here. . . . / We few, we
happy few, we band of brothers."[11] More succinctly, Rabbi (Captain US
Navy Chaplain Corps, retired) Irv Elson quoted that beautiful Hebrew
phrase of shared experience that many veterans have with one another:
"*Hameivin yavin*—those who understand will understand."[12]

As Reform rabbis, we have a sacred obligation to guide our *talmidim*
(students) from the time of bet mitzvah through confirmation and high
school graduation to live lives of selfless service. Again and again, we
must inspire them with the hallowed words of President Kennedy, "Ask
not what your country can do for you. Ask what you can do for your
country."[13] We must teach them according to the words of Isaiah and
Ben Azzai. We must remind them of the deeds of the heroes who came
before them—the firefighters of 9/11, the soldiers who stormed the
beaches of Normandy and liberated Dachau, and the heroes of Lexington, Concord, Valley Forge, and Yorktown. And as they prepare to leave
home and we bless them with *T'filat HaDerech* (the Traveler's Prayer), we
should do so knowing that we have encouraged them to embark on lives
of altruistic service and noble volunteerism, whether that means giving
their blood to accident victims or cancer patients, providing canned
goods and old coats to the homeless, donating their time as drivers for
Meals on Wheels, becoming a paramedic, EMT, firefighter, or police
officer in their community, or serving in the military. The United
States, this noble experiment of democracy, will only live on if the next

generation puts on the camouflage uniform—the immortal cloak of service—as their parents, grandparents, great-grandparents, and all those who came before them did.

Perhaps President Ronald Reagan said it best: "Freedom is a fragile thing and it's never more than one generation away from extinction. It is not ours by way of inheritance; it must be fought for and defended constantly by each generation, for it comes only once to a people."[14]

Serving in the military is not an easy life, a convenient life, or a safe life, but it is a calling that ensures the preservation of our freedom and the conservation of our way of life. This country has given us as Jews so much. Serving in uniform is one of the best ways Jews can say "thank you" to America and, in my experience, is a truly effective Jewish response to trauma.

Notes

1. "Recognition of US Liberating Army Units," *Holocaust Encyclopedia*, United States Holocaust Memorial Museum, https://encyclopedia.ushmm.org/content/en/article/us-army-units.

2. As translated in *Mishkan T'filah for Gatherings*, ed. Elyse D. Frishman and Sue Ann Wasserman (CCAR Press, 2009), 113.

3. "National Guard Heritage Paintings," National Guard, https://www.nationalguard.mil/Resources/Image-Gallery/Historical-Paintings/Heritage-Paintings/.

4. Clayton R. Newell, *The Regular Army Before the Civil War: 1845–1860*, CMH Pub 75-1 (Washington, DC: United States Army Center of Military History, 2014), 51, https://history.army.mil/html/books/075/75-1/CMH_Pub_75-1.pdf; Gian Gentile et al., *The Evolution of U.S. Military Policy from the Constitution to the Present*, vol. 1, *The Old Regime: The Army, Militia, and Volunteers from Colonial Times to the Spanish-American War* (RAND, 2020), https://www.rand.org/pubs/research_reports/RR1995z1.html.

5. "Texas National Guard to Help El Paso Morgues with Virus Dead," *Associated Press News*, November 21, 2020, https://www.apnews.com/article/el-paso-coronavirus-pandemic-texas-greg-abbott-3c66b17b93614c-be4ea24689bb643c4b.

6. Michael J. Carden, "Minnesota Guard to Command Active-Duty Forces in Iraq," National Guard, December 11, 2008, https://www.nationalguard.mil/News/Article-View/Article/573677/minnesota-guard-to-command-active-duty-forces-in-iraq/.

7. Darron Salzer, "Post 9/11: This Isn't Your Father's National Guard,"

National Guard, September 9, 2010, https://www.nationalguard.mil/News/Article-View/Article/576443/post-911-this-isnt-your-fathers-national-guard/.

8. Erich B. Smith, "Guard's Global Reach, Capabilities Support National Defense Strategy," National Guard, December 5, 2022, https://www.nationalguard.mil/News/Article/3236186/guards-global-reach-capabilities-support-national-defense-strategy/.

9. Katherine Schaeffer, "The Changing Face of America's Veteran Population," Pew Research Center, November 8, 2023, https://www.pewresearch.org/short-reads/2023/11/08/the-changing-face-of-americas-veteran-population/.

10. Military OneSource, https://www.militaryonesource.mil/; "Combat and Operational Stress Control," Military Health System, https://health.mil/Military-Health-Topics/Centers-of-Excellence/Psychological-Health-Center-of-Excellence/Psychological-Health-Readiness/Combat-and-Operational-Stress-Control; "Master Resilience Training," United States Army, https://www.armyresilience.army.mil/ard/R2/Master-Resilience-Training.html; "Building Strong & Ready Teams," United States Army, https://bsrt.army.mil/; Yellow Ribbon Reintegration Program, https://www.yellowribbon.mil/.

11. William Shakespeare, *Henry V*, act 4, scene 3, lines 66–67, 62.

12. "Honoring our Veterans: Service and Sacrifice," Washington National Cathedral, https://www.youtube.com/watch?v=NnQtoQQsjQk&t=76s.

13. John Fitzgerald Kennedy, "Presidential Inaugural Address," United States Archives, January 20, 1961, https://www.archives.gov/milestone-documents/president-john-f-kennedys-inaugural-address.

14. Ronald Reagan, "California Gubernatorial Address, January 5, 1967," Ronald Reagan Presidential Library & Museum, https://www.reaganlibrary.gov/archives/speech/january-5-1967-inaugural-address-public-ceremony.

20

The Holocaust and October 7
The Personal Impact of Generational Trauma

RABBI DAVID SPINRAD

Don't look back. Something may be gaining on you.
—*Satchel Paige*[1]

ALL MY LIFE, I've tried to stay out in front of something without realizing what I was doing. I didn't even know what "it" was. After agreeing to write a chapter on the Holocaust for this book, I regretted that decision and resisted starting it. I now understand why: If I slow down, if I stop, if I look back, the darkness that has been gaining might overtake me. October 7, 2023, and the subsequent antisemitism dislodged my suppressed intergenerational trauma and brought it to the surface. I am not okay.

Growing up as the first-born grandson of survivors, the Holocaust was always present. Lurking. A weight that was never spoken about. My grandfather died when I was seven. I never got to ask him about what he experienced. When I was thirteen, I asked my grandmother. I can still see her jaw tighten and her lips purse. Wordlessly, she gave me such a look of finality that I knew to never ask again. My mother never knew what happened to our family. My auntie doesn't know what happened. In Israel, I asked my grandmother's nephew. He was a little boy and somehow survived as a very young child. He only remembered wanting to make the adults happy and that talking about the past made them sad.

My family not talking about the Holocaust taught me to not talk about the Holocaust. In the absence of details and understanding of where I came from, my Holocaust stories became an amalgamation of the collective nightmare. A girlfriend once said to me that since the stories of my ancestors were lost, maybe the Nazis won. That woman has been gone from my life for twenty-five years, but the pain of her words never left.

To compensate for the unspoken weight I carried, to balance the burden of the intergenerational trauma, I chose strength. I chose to be a defender of our people, to be so strong that no one could hurt me or us. I excelled in sports and in fitness, dispelling the stereotype of the weak Jew who went like a lamb to the slaughter. I chose to be driven toward excellence, suffering endlessly my mistakes and dismissing my successes. I thought that if I was perfect, nothing could get to me. I chose vigilance, anticipating every possible outcome so nothing bad could happen again. I chose the enormous responsibility of being a leader of the Jewish people, embracing my duty to serve not only the Jewish people of today, but vowing to honor our ancestors of yesterday and inspire our descendants of tomorrow. I chose Zionism, the right of the Jewish people to self-determination and self-defense in our indigenous, ancestral homeland. God forbid it should ever happen again, we would be safe there. And because loyalty mattered above all else, when we argued about Israel, we kept it to ourselves. Division to the outside world meant vulnerability. Thankfully, I also chose laughter. My mom stuffing our cupboards so full of canned food that the doors would not close became a dark "if you know, you know" source of humor. But it also expressed her trauma.

It would be untrue to say I chose my wife because she, too, is the grandchild of survivors. However, to the people who understand, about her I offer the highest praise: She is the kind of person who would come up with an extra potato for our family if we were locked in the ghetto.

What I inherited genetically and learned from my upbringing gave me some of my best attributes: strength, drive, vigilance, responsibility, loyalty, a sense of humor. All of these traits helped me achieve success. But because they originated at least partly as trauma responses, my attributes are overdeveloped and unbalanced, to protect me from the darkness. October 7 and the aftermath from which I write these words is the first time this became evident to me.

I was forty-two when I first heard the idea that vulnerability and weakness are not synonymous. I still don't necessarily believe it. Other than my family and a few friends I can count on one hand (with fingers left over), I don't fully trust people. And when it comes to forgiveness, the best I can offer is to forgive and remember. To forgive and forget might be dangerous. Most of all, inside of me lurks the fear that something terrible will happen. I remember my mom once said that she always felt like she was waiting for the other shoe to drop. When she said that, I felt relieved: If she felt the way I felt, then how I felt must be normal. But normal meant that no matter how strong and vigilant and responsible I was—the other shoe would inevitably drop. Normal meant expecting that bad things would eventually happen. It meant that evil would again turn its face toward the Jews. My scorecard was always nearby, ready to keep a tally of those who stood with us, those who stood against us, and those who stood idly by.

October 7 and its aftermath were defining moments—moments when I understood where everyone stood for me. Antisemitism was illuminated, and my understanding of antisemitism shifted from something I associated with the far right (for example, white supremacists, Christian nationalists, and neo-Nazis) to something that is associated as well with the far left. I saw that antisemitism has no political affiliation. Rather, it is a systemic pillar of Western civilization, contending that Jews are the locus of evil in the world. Whatever is most detestable in a given place and time becomes inevitably Jewish. When we dig down deep enough, we find that we are hated for our very existence.

Today, Israel and Zionism have become proxies for hatred against the Jewish people. Being an anti-Zionist champion of Palestinian liberation is the cause de rigueur for some people. Against the Jewish state and without an iota of intellectual honesty, behind kaffiyehs worn both as identity politics fashion statements and to protect the anonymity of activists whom I believe are too cowardly to show their faces, absurd, hurtful accusations of racism, white settler colonialism, apartheid, and genocide are the norm. "Zionist" has become an epithet. In cities and on campuses across the West, protestors menacingly chant, "There is only one solution, intifada, revolution," "From the River to the Sea, Palestine will be free," "We don't want no two-state, we want 1948," and "Hezbollah, Hezbollah, kill another Zionist now."[2] When that illuminating flare finally fell from the sky, it landed with a thud—not unlike the sound of the other shoe dropping.

As I reread my words, I sense my defensiveness. The attributes by which I define myself and those I trust the most are on high alert. But why would I not emphasize and lead with my strength, vigilance, and responsibility when the Jewish people are under attack? This feels like the defining moment of my life. Why shouldn't I take a defensive stance when the presidents of Harvard, MIT, and Penn said, "It depends on the context," when asked if it was against their respective university codes of conduct to call for the genocide of Jews? Why wouldn't I speak up in outrage when UN Women waited fifty-five days to condemn the brutal attacks by Hamas or when the #MeToo movement ignored the sexual violence by Hamas against Israeli women? How can I not voice my anger when Jews are barred (couched as "Zionists prohibited") from businesses and when we are blocked from public spaces, when our horror is met with cold silence by those who are unaffected?[3] What am I supposed to do with my sadness when what is being perpetuated against Jews would never be acceptable if targeted at other marginalized communities? Why would I not act from my understanding that "Never Again" is now?

I am not so trusting of the world right now. This is the loneliest I have ever felt. In my devotion to Israel and my outspokenness against Islamic fundamentalists—who willingly sacrifice their own civilians, even their own children, and who openly express their desire to eradicate the State of Israel and eliminate the Jewish people worldwide—I have lost people I thought were my friends and professional relationships with those I once counted as allies. I am fine with that.

And yet, being perpetually on high alert has taken its toll. I am weary. Even though there is abundant evidence that the Jewish people are under assault, not everything that happens confirms this belief. I'm only choosing to believe that it does. Sometimes silence from neighbors or local Christian pastors just means Israel and the war are not on their minds like it is on mine. Intellectually I know that what I am seeing on social media and hearing on the news is not fully representative of everyone, everywhere, and is designed to stir my anger and fear, triggering my trauma response and initiating this endless cycle.

I do not want to keep feeling the way I am feeling, but I am afraid. I am afraid that the world will again abandon the Jews and turn a blind eye to existential wars against Israel. I am afraid to give anything less than 100 percent in my people's hour of need. I am afraid to fail in my responsibility and loyalty as a leader. I am afraid that if I am not strong and defensive, rejective of vulnerability, always trying to be the best and do the best, that a load-bearing wall in my constructed identity might crumble. I would collapse. Most of all, I am afraid to be afraid. There is no room for it.

What do I do? October 7 and its ongoing aftermath activated painful, intergenerational trauma. While I knew it was there, I never identified it this way before. Writing this essay forced me to confront the darkness that has overtaken me. Here, I share for the first time the agonizing ways I am personally experiencing this terrible war and its impact on me, because of what I inherited and what I was taught by my family.

But I know I can't go on like this forever. I need to talk to someone. I need to talk to a trauma-informed therapist. I need to be in a safe and quiet space with someone who can help me to find my way forward on a path that is unknown and scary without abandoning all the gifts that make me, *me*.

Last, I need to know my actual family story. I'm staggering trying to hold the abstraction of our collective history of oppression and persecution as my own. I need the story to be smaller. Specific. Even in the most terrible details, knowing where it happened and when it happened and to whom it happened might help to heal this wound in my soul.

Writing this chapter was difficult and painful. But I am hopeful that somehow my own struggles will in some small measure be helpful to others. The Holocaust has never been something that can be summarized in a chapter, and perhaps the emotional impact of October 7 cannot be either. But still, we try. Still, I try. It is true that I am not okay. But maybe that's okay too.

NOTES

1. Scott Pitoniak, "In 1971, Satchel Paige Came to Cooperstown," National Baseball Hall of Fame, https://baseballhall.org/discover/in-1971-satchel-paige-came-to-cooperstown.

2. Judith Shulevitz, "Listen to What They're Chanting," *The Atlantic*, May 8, 2024, https://www.theatlantic.com/books/archive/2024/05/pro-palestinian-protests-columbia-chants/678321/.

3. See Jory Rand, "Jewish UC Santa Barbara Students Fear for Safety After Antisemitic Signs Appear on Campus," *ABC 7 Eyewitness News*, Febru-

ary 27, 2024, https://abc7.com/uc-santa-barbara-antisemitic-signs-multicultural-center-instagram-anti-zionist/14474548/; Marcy Oster, "Toronto Restaurant Loses Business Deals After Saying 'Zionists' Not Welcome," *The Times of Israel*, July 9, 2024, https://www.timesofisrael.com/toronto-restaurant-loses-business-deals-after-saying-zionists-not-welcome/; and Trevor Myers, "Jewish Community Condemns SLC Bar After Bar Declares 'No Zionists Allowed,'" *Wasatch Front News*, ABC4.com, March 6, 2024, https://www.abc4.com/news/wasatch-front/jewish-community-condemns-slc-bar-after-bar-declares-no-zionists-allowed/.

21

Witnessing History

A Memphis Rabbi's Journey Through the
Assassination of Reverend Dr. Martin Luther King Jr.

RABBI HARRY K. DANZIGER

IT IS AUGUST 1964, and I am the new young assistant rabbi in Memphis. I am scheduled to drive to Clarksdale, Mississippi, for a regional temple youth meeting. I say to a congregant, half-jokingly, "Maybe I should change my Ohio license plate before I go." He says, not at all jokingly, "You sure should!" A rabbi with Ohio plates on a Mississippi highway in 1964 could be in real danger.

I was born and raised in a segregated world in West Virginia. It was unremarkable to me that one never saw African Americans in a restaurant we went to. Schools were segregated, though I was in high school when *Brown v. Board of Education* declared segregation unconstitutional. West Virginia did not race to comply, but neither was there the angry defiance or outright violence that marked the Deep South.

The famous "temple bombing" had occurred in Atlanta some years before. A prominent Cleveland rabbi was brutally beaten in Hattiesburg. A few years later, both the temple and the rabbi's home in Jackson, Mississippi, would be bombed. It was more than a little traumatic to realize that in 1964 an Ohio license plate and the title "rabbi" could be dangerous, if not deadly.

It is April 1968, and I am now an associate rabbi in Memphis. We are about to leave our apartment to go to the annual Greek Festival at the Greek Orthodox Church. The news bulletin announces that Dr. Martin Luther King Jr. has been shot and killed only a few miles away. That night, American cities burn with fires set by angry, grieving people. But not Memphis. In Memphis, the Black community is stunned, frightened, and immediately subject to a curfew and an overwhelming police presence.

The next morning, I join a number of Memphis clergy for a service in memory of MLK and then a march to the mayor's office. When I arrive at the cathedral, the first person I meet is Reverend James Lawson. Lawson was a close associate of Dr. King and, in many ways, the chief strategist and theorist of nonviolence. I knew him only slightly. What do I say to him? He has lost a personal friend, and his people have lost their prophet. How do I express meaningful sympathies? I think I mumbled something about being sorry, inadequate though it might be. I realize now that Rabbi Shimon ben Elazar was right. "Do not console [your fellow] while their dead lies before them" (*Pirkei Avot* 4:23).

At the cathedral, we call for an end to the sanitation strike, a strike where the signature signs workers carried said "I am a man." Memphis—where progress had come peacefully in integrating public facilities and the like—was coming face-to-face with the abject poverty and exploitation that many in the Black community encountered daily. We march to the mayor's office, where my senior colleague rebukes the mayor on behalf of all the clergy assembled there.

The strike eventually ends with a salary increase, union recognition, and improved labor conditions. But Memphis is forever changed. We who spoke of "a wonderful place for families" or who recalled that Memphis means "place of good abode" had come face-to-face with conditions many of us had previously ignored.

Dallas was the scene of the assassination of John F. Kennedy and Los Angeles of his brother Robert. But neither of those cities is so identified with the tragedy there as is Memphis with the murder of Dr. King. Memphis was characterized by responsible mainstream media as the embodiment of the worst of Southern segregation and bigotry. *Time* magazine famously called it a "Southern backwater" and a "decaying Mississippi River town." Though MLK was apparently killed by someone who had simply tracked him to Memphis, the stain on the city became indelible. It was as if the city were an accomplice to the murder.

On the Sunday after the assassination, Memphians—white and Black—fill a stadium under the banner "Memphis Cares." It is the expression of a city forced to face its own ugly side and imagine better. Fears about violence at this first interracial gathering prove to be unfounded. I go to the event also worried for what might happen. I am on the platform to offer a prayer rather than my senior colleague, Rabbi

James Wax, who received death threats after he confronted the mayor for his role in prolonging the strike. These death threats have a personal impact. For some time following the assassination, I remain apprehensive for Rabbi Wax. In a time when we have no "active shooter drills," a time when churches and synagogues are bombed but not attacked with guns, I always keep my eyes on the doors at the rear of the sanctuary when he is at the lectern. What I would do in the event of violence I don't know, but my instinctive fear is a measure of the reality of this time and place.

Still, it was important to show that Memphis cared about the revered high school principal who told me, "Rabbi, to you I'm Dr., with my degrees from universities, but on the street I'm just another [n-word]." It was important to say that Memphis cared about those who had fought for civil rights—Black and white—who faced death threats. It was a way to say that Memphis cared about the formerly forgotten sanitation workers marching with signs saying "I am a man."

April 1968 is long past, but as is true of many who survive cancer, all is not over when one is cancer-free. Some experience the suspense of periodic blood tests, scopes, or other diagnostics. Like a patient who has heard a diagnosis of cancer, a city once traumatized will never be the same.

That weekend my wife and I see a Jeep with several armed National Guardsmen on it. I am almost thirty years old. My wife, Jeanne, is twenty-two. It is our first time seeing troops in the streets of our city. We think of our nephews, ages twelve and fourteen, who are seeing this, and we think of the child Jeanne is carrying. We often speak of things passed *l'dor vador*, "from generation to generation." We realized even then that we were passing on a world different from the one we took for granted.

The Monday following the assassination, a friend and I walk to City Hall Plaza for a memorial to Dr. King. The streets are virtually empty. We come to a corner where we would normally cross, and a young National Guardsman with a rifle and fixed bayonet says, "I'm sorry, gentlemen, but you'll have to go to the next corner."

The Sunday after the assassination is model seder day at religious school. At each of the class seders I play a portion of MLK's "I Have a Dream" speech. I want the children to have some understanding of what has happened and to whom. How can one have Pesach 1968 without noting the death of the very prophet of freedom in our city?

After 1968, we would have to constantly confront the "zero-sum game" mentality that inaccurately assumes that what is good for one race automatically costs the other. And we would face all the problems of cities where large minority populations lived in poverty.

Memphians' ongoing trauma has many facets shared with society at large. The wealth gap between Black and white communities remains deep, but much has been done to answer basic human needs. Greater Black presence at every level of government has made a huge difference—both cosmetic and substantive—but racism persists through too much of our nation.

More than half a century after the assassination, we know that "Memphis Cares" was more than a bumper sticker or a public relations slogan. In the wake of the assassination, a small group of clergy and laypeople formed what may first sound like just another place for discussing religious similarities and differences. The Metropolitan Inter-Faith Association grew out of a need not to change laws, but to change lives. It was a response to the traumatic truth that those who lived in poverty could not wait for government programs and legislation to ease their lives. Before the term "food insecurity" was coined, there were hungry people. Before "homeless" gave way to "unhoused" or "curbside community," there were those who slept in doorways.

MIFA, as it came to be known, committed itself to addressing the immediate needs that plagued individuals and families in Memphis. While others undertook the mission to change laws and still others the task of changing hearts, MIFA's mission was to answer everyday needs for real people.

Many Memphians were committed to Hillel's dictum, "If I am for myself alone, what am I?" MIFA echoed the third part of Hillel's dictum: "If not now, when?" (*Pirkei Avot* 1:14).

Religious liberals and conservatives, people of faith and no faith, were drawn to involve themselves in this agency. Its mission was, quite simply, to change living conditions in the here and now. It was hands-on and face-to-face with those in the greatest need. Eventually

MIFA would address hunger, shelter, job training, emergency services, clothing, utilities aid, and senior care issues. It became the largest community service agency in the region. It received support in the form of volunteers and funding from a vast array of congregations and individuals, many of whom had little in common with each other except for a commitment to making "Memphis Cares" real.

Over the years, much has changed in Memphis. But many of us still remember those plaintive signs that said "I am a man" and the terrible images of those days. For some, the response has been to try to change the world at large. Others try to change the community one life at a time. When the obstacles seem daunting, we try to respond in the spirit of Rabbi Tarfon, who said, "You are not required to complete the task, but neither are you free to desist from it" (*Pirkei Avot* 2:21).

22

September 11, 2001

Crossing the Narrow Bridge

Rabbi Serge A. Lippe

T UESDAY, SEPTEMBER 11, 2001, began with a crisp, clear, azure-blue morning. There wasn't a single cloud in the sky over Brooklyn, not that that was the first thing on our minds as my wife, Deb, and I walked over to Congregation Mount Sinai (the local Conservative synagogue and polling place) on Cadman Plaza to cast our votes in the New York City mayoral primary.

We had lived in our Brooklyn neighborhood for just over four years, and September 11 was the start of my fifth High Holy Day season on the pulpit of Brooklyn Heights Synagogue (BHS). The main thing on my mind that morning was our synagogue's preparations for Rosh HaShanah, which we would observe at Plymouth Church of the Pilgrims in six days, on Monday evening, September 17.

Making the short walk from our co-op on Pierrepont Street, we were hoping to avoid the longer late-morning voting lines so that each of us could make it to our offices in a timely manner. As we entered Congregation Mount Sinai, we heard someone comment that a Cessna had flown into one of the towers of the World Trade Center (WTC). The idea of a small prop plane hitting one of the towers didn't seem totally beyond the pale. As we exited the voting center some fifteen minutes later, we now heard about a second plane hitting the Twin Towers. We didn't yet know they were commercial jetliners. But we knew that two planes hitting the WTC towers in a short window eight years after the terrorist bombing in the WTC basement likely meant another attack. Friends, colleagues, and members of our congregation worked in the towers. We were hoping it wasn't as bad as it seemed, as bad as we feared.

We walked the four blocks to the Brooklyn Heights Promenade, which sits above the Brooklyn-Queens Expressway and provides a wide, cobbled, half-kilometer pedestrian vista of Lower Manhattan and beyond, from the Brooklyn Bridge to the north to the Verrazzano-Narrows

Bridge to the south. There wasn't a cloud in that perfect blue sky, but two streams of smoke were billowing, one from each of the Twin Towers. At that distance, it was hard to estimate the size of the impacts, hard to gauge the degree of destruction, and hard to imagine the deaths that had already just happened—much less those that would follow.

Under that morning's high-pressure system, the winds carried papers from offices in the towers across the East River to land in the calmer surroundings of Brooklyn. It was surreal. This gorgeous day—now heavy with fear and dread.

Deb's first inclination was to get to work at Morgan Stanley Dean Witter (MSDW). A technologist in the financial world, she worked primarily at MSDW in midtown, but back in 2001 she also had a standing weekly meeting at the equity trading floor in the WTC South Tower. At the time, MSDW was the largest tenant of the WTC, with thirty-five floors distributed across towers one, two, and five.

Deb's inclination to get to work momentarily set off my own sense of panic. "What the hell are you thinking?" I thought, as images of my wife putting life and limb at risk below ground flashed by nightmarishly—if only momentarily—in my imagination. But by 9:15 a.m. there was no way to get from Brooklyn to Manhattan; the New York City subway system was completely shut down. Street traffic had also ground to a halt. By 9:45 a.m. TV and radio informed us that all air travel had been suspended nationally.

We took refuge at home. At 9:59 a.m. we watched on television as the South Tower collapsed. At 10:28 a.m. the North Tower collapsed. That wasn't supposed to happen. We knew from Deb's dad, an internationally regarded forensic concrete engineer, that the WTC towers had been built with the assurance that fire wouldn't take them down. But no one had planned for commercial airplanes filled with jet fuel exploding into them like rockets.

Fortunately, MSDW's director of security at the WTC, Rick Rescorla, had anticipated further attacks after 1993 and that morning activated the evacuation procedures he had set in place. Rick evacuated 2,687 MSDW employees. Thirteen MSDW employees died that day, including Rick. He died going back into the South Tower to help evacuate more people.

The securities firm of Cantor Fitzgerald had its headquarters in the North Tower, between the 101st and 105th floors, immediately above where American Airlines flight 11 struck. All 658 employees in the tower that morning were killed, the largest loss for any company that day. One of those employees was also forty-seven-year-old BHS member Catherine Chirls,[1] wife and mother, who worked with eSpeed, Cantor Fitzgerald's electronic trading platform.

Other members of the BHS community had, like Deb and me, gone to vote that morning and delayed their travel to offices in the Twin Towers and Lower Manhattan. It was still the era of flip phones and Blackberries, but with the fall of the towers and their antennas, it was dedicated landlines that were now ringing off the hook with voices on the other end of the line asking if we were safe and if we were home.

Yes, *we* were safe, *we* were home, but there were too many people we couldn't be sure were. Worry and guilt weighed on me almost physically as we watched and listened.

In 2001, network and cable television news and AM radio news reports still ruled the fastest flow of information. We soon heard the reports about the attack on the Pentagon and the downing of United Airlines flight 93 in Pennsylvania.

Anxiety and agitation mixed with profound sadness and confusion—emotions that smothered my own usually sharp sensibilities. A jumble of incoherent questions kept popping up in my head: Were we safe? Was this attack over? What should I be doing? Who did we know who might not make it home today?

In the immediate aftermath, we opened the BHS sanctuary to the community to serve as a gathering place, called our home-limited members, offered evening services each day, and began to rethink what the Days of Awe would be like as security around synagogues in NYC went beyond anything we had ever experienced. Several thousand New York State National Guardsmen would flood NYC alongside the NYPD over the next forty-eight hours. There were literally guns and armored vehicles moving through the city, not to mention Air Force jets thundering overhead. NYC had become an active military site, and the sight of soldiers in uniform and heavy weapons, rather than reassuring, added to my own sense of anxiety and insecurity.

Within that same time period, I heard from clergy colleagues from our local interfaith association. Was everyone accounted for, how could we support one another, what families needed special attention? Reaching out to members and neighbors gave me something meaningful and steadying to do. It didn't feel sufficient, but it was something. It helped me push most of the doubt and worry aside.

Within days, we gathered on the Brooklyn Heights Promenade— this time as a community of churches, synagogues, and our one local mosque. We spoke up as religious leaders against hate and terror, offering prayers, songs, and chants in English, Hebrew, and Arabic. We sounded the shofar. We did our best to acknowledge our collective loss and grief, fear and anger. The anger came last, but it came—from those of us who experienced the unfamiliar combination of fear and powerlessness.

The trauma of 9/11 came not from one direction but from many. There was the loss of friends and colleagues, mentors and protégés who perished in the towers, some of whom initially remained unaccounted for. The survivors who had escaped the towers and surrounding neighborhoods carried the sensory overload of the experience with them. For youngsters shielded from the worst, there were still the friends and classmates whose parents did not come home that day. We dealt with the displacement of members who had lived in Lower Manhattan. There were deep fears of a repeat attack. There were many funerals and shivah services without body or burial for closure. At times, I was drawn back to the emotions of a decade earlier when I started my career, feeling like a professional imposter. Who was I to guide and comfort and reassure those dealing with such profound loss and tragedy? But whatever my doubts, the need was there, and I pushed my own reservations aside to do the work.

In the first days after 9/11, NYC was eerily silent. There was still the unabated smell of smoke in the air of Brooklyn Heights and barely any traffic on the street. It was a reserved NYC that was still reeling. New Yorkers were unusually polite and thoughtful, but also walking on eggshells. We didn't know what might set off a proverbial aftershock for someone else. We were cautious with one another in a way that I had never experienced before. Personally, it wasn't just that I was concerned about accidentally setting someone off—it was also the fear of unintentionally loosening the ties that were holding my own somewhat fragile balance together.

Like every other rabbi in the country, I filed away my original Rosh HaShanah sermon and started writing from scratch. But what to say? So many of our members had lost friends, colleagues, and acquaintances. I knew we needed something closer to a eulogy than a sermon, but not quite that either. Years of song leading in high school, college, and rabbinical school had taught me that sometimes song has more power than words alone. I knew I would not be the only colleague invoking the "narrow bridge" we were all standing on that evening.

Rabbi Baruch Chait composed the song "Kol HaOlam Kulo Gesher Tzar M'od" while performing for Israeli soldiers during the Yom Kippur War. The song is usually translated as "The entire world is but a narrow bridge; the most important thing is not to be afraid at all."[2] It is based on the teaching of Reb Nachman of Bratzlav, who wrote in his *Likutei Moharan*: *V'da, shehaadam tzarich laavor al gesher tzar m'od m'od, v'hak'lal v'ha-ikar shelo yitpacheid k'lal*, "And know, that a person needs to cross a very, very narrow bridge, and the essential principle is not to make yourself entirely afraid."[3]

Reb Nachman's original text is slightly different from the words of Rabbi Chait's song, but the difference is important. You couldn't sensibly expect anyone in NYC during those days "not to be afraid at all." But not to make oneself *more* afraid, not to add to one's existing fear, not to give into the terror of that time—that seemed to be wisdom that I could share on this Rosh HaShanah.

The core of Reb Nachman's message isn't about denying fear. It is about not allowing fear to freeze us in place. His words remind us that life is lived by moving forward, by not allowing ourselves to become immobilized.

As we gathered for worship, it was clear that attendance at our Erev Rosh HaShanah service at Plymouth Church of the Pilgrims filled the historic church's pews. I saw faces of members I had never once seen inside the synagogue (or at Plymouth for the holy days). There were also members of the larger community joining us, seeking the anchor and stability of neighbors and maybe even the reassurance of the Divine.

We began services by singing Rabbi Chait's melody. I'm not sure how long we sang together, but it was a good while. Not every set of lips was moving, but I think every one of us felt caught up in the power of that song. Connected and reflective. Exercising spiritual muscles that had been locked and rigid for the past week.

There at Plymouth Church—our long-standing "home for the holy days"—it felt as though I was really *seeing* the community. Looking backward and looking forward, I saw all those around me supporting one another—each in their own struggle, each offering their own effort.

Our collective song and voices unlocked the recognition that for the past six days we had been standing on a precipice and that up until that moment we had been holding our individual and collective breath. The "bridge" might be very narrow, but we were making it a little bit wider, making room for others to stand alongside us.

Our song opened up a space, at least for me, to momentarily peek or even peer over the side of the bridge, to recognize my own fear rather than deny it, which is what I had been doing for the past six days.

I could not move forward, I could not grieve, and I certainly could not comfort or lead if I remained locked in place denying, avoiding my own fear, pain, and loss. None of us can. Singing that song, I realized: We were in this together.

My fears were real, but now acknowledged and shared with those who would help me—even as I helped them cross the bridge.

NOTES

1. "Catherine Ellen Chirls: A Mother's Presence," *New York Times*, https://archive.nytimes.com/www.nytimes.com/library/national/met_MISSING_1004_chirls.html.
2. Adapted translation from *Mishkan T'filah: A Reform Siddur* (CCAR Press, 2007), 643.
3. Nachman of Bratzlav, *Likutei Moharan* 2:48:2:7. Translated by the author. See https://www.sefaria.org/Likutei_Moharan%2C_Part_II.48.2.1.

23

Two Bombs

How the Boston Marathon Bombing
Changed My Life

R ABBI B ENJAMIN D AVID

T HOSE TWO BOMBS changed my life. Before I get to that, I need to explain the hours that preceded the bombs.

When you stand on the starting line of the Boston Marathon, emotion surges in your veins. You feel in your heart the weight of everything to come. There is anxiety. There is hope. There is fear. There is appreciation that you made it to this impossible, iconic place at last. There is the knowledge that this race—over a century old, 26.2 miles long, and riddled with rolling hills—has challenged and propelled countless runners to be at their absolute best. It's more than a marathon; it's a question: Who are you? That's what the Boston Marathon asked me that fateful day: Who are you?

This was my first Boston Marathon. Training had gone well—weeks upon weeks of early-morning runs, long runs on the weekend, eating to fuel my body, and trying to fine-tune my mindset. I did all of this while I balanced the responsibilities of being a senior rabbi, husband, and father to three young children. My trusty running partner, Rabbi Scott Weiner, was participating in the marathon with me. He and I had run marathons along a good portion of the East Coast. We were tried and tested, but Boston is something else. The Boston Marathon is about history and heritage. It has defined and redefined runners for over a century. The expectations are different. The runners all around are different. We felt all of it.

Just before the race began, I called on a quote from Isaiah, that we should "run and not be weary" (40:31). It was time to find out what the day had in store.

The first half of the race was relatively uneventful. The route guides runners downhill for a good portion. There is temptation to believe that things are going better than anticipated. This is how the Boston course lures runners in and tempts them to abandon their race plan. Wise runners know better. Scott and I held back as much as possible.

About halfway through, we passed through the town of Wellesley and the iconic Wellesley "scream tunnel," made up of raucous college students out in full force to cheer on the runners. It comes as a boost at a time when most runners (myself included) feel the pain of the miles starting to accumulate. My legs were getting heavy to be sure. Just past mile seventeen, there is a sweeping right at a fire station and the beginning of the infamous Newton Hills, those relentless rollers that are so much a part of the Boston Marathon. The climbing culminates just past mile twenty with the notorious Heartbreak Hill, which has decimated the ambitions of so many.

I tried to keep calm. I tried to keep breathing. The pain was real now. I climbed and climbed, my legs burning. My back ached. I felt it in my shoulders, in my hands, behind my eyes. Somehow, I made it to the final stretch of the race, past Fenway Park on my right and the Citgo sign that signals one mile to go. A right on Hereford and left on Boylston and I was finally (finally!) in sight of the finish. After all the preparation, the countless dreams I had of this exact moment, the people I carried in my heart, the sheer sense of love I felt for my family and a benevolent God up above, there it was—the finish line of the Boston Marathon.

I ran past the line with my arms raised. I was elated and exhausted. It was over. We did it. With medals around our necks, Scott and I began our short walk to the hotel. We were delirious and proud. We hobbled. We recounted the race to each other. We rubbed shoulders with hundreds of other runners, accents mixing with emotions and the humility the course had cast on all of us.

We were less than a block away from the finish line when we heard an extremely loud BOOM. Everyone stopped where they were. Car crash? A collapsed bleacher? Something at a construction site? Then another BOOM. We looked around, unsure. We kept walking. Then, after a minute, came the first wave of ambulances and police cars. Someone went hustling by: "Two bombs exploded at the finish line."

My mind whirred. I knew that this marathon, forever predicated on life, humanity, and the enduring strength of the human spirit, had changed in an instant. The Boston Marathon stood for all of that. Now it would stand for something else.

On weary legs, we hurried to our hotel room and crowded around the TV. I reached out to my wife to let her know I was okay. My phone buzzed with concerned family and friends. Outside the window, we watched officers frantically clear the area and attend to the injured. Everyone feared more attacks were imminent. With our aching legs and foggy minds, we considered what to do next.

However, there was nothing to do and nowhere to go. After running twenty-six miles, our bodies were starved for food and drink, yet the city was quickly shutting down. We wanted to be with loved ones, but we were far from home. We were in a place of profound limbo and uncertainty—stuck in front of the television, wondering what would come next.

After a sleepless night, I began my long drive home. I had experienced a truly devastating and horrifying event. In the end, three people died that April day, seventeen people lost limbs, and countless others were injured. During the drive, I repeatedly considered that it could have been me. Was it fate or luck or something else that had me just a few hundred feet away and not directly at the site of the blasts? What did it mean? Would this change who I was as a husband, as a dad, as a rabbi, as a marathoner? Would it change who I was as a Jew? Undoubtedly, the answer to all of it would be "yes."

As the weeks passed, I continued to mull over the kind of indelible mark the day would leave. With the terrorists now accounted for, I could think clearly about what I had survived. Rather than move in the direction of anger at a world that felt so violent and unforgiving, I found myself feeling more and more thankful that I was alive. I actively refused to go where Job went, when he proclaimed, "God has deprived me of justice; God has embittered me" (Job 27:2). Rather, I thanked God that my story would continue. I began to work consciously—in study, in prayer, while out running—at living with a grateful heart. I considered the words of our tradition: "Adonai I praise with all my heart; all Your wonders will I in tales recount" (Psalm 9:2). Surviving the bombings meant I could commit myself even more vigorously to my work, aligning myself with the hurting and being there for those in pain. I vowed to live in tribute to those three souls whose lives were cut short. I remained anxious around crowds for a time and less than eager to sign up for another big-city race. In time, however, after overcoming cancer just a few years later, I returned to the Boston Marathon. I ran the race in 2017, a kind of triumphant reclaiming of those famed streets.

As time passed, I settled more and more firmly into this place of thankfulness. It became easier to do, perhaps because of my being steadfast about it day after day. I thought often about the words of the Psalmist: "God is my helper, the sustainer of my soul. . . . God delivered me out of trouble" (Psalm 54:6, 9). Increasingly, this felt like the appropriate place to put my life-altering experiences—not in victimhood or bitterness, but in abundant presence and faith. This is where I choose to dwell.

24

A Personal and Communal Journey Toward Healing

The Story of Parkland

RABBI MELISSA ZALKIN STOLLMAN

IMAGINE SMALL-TOWN suburban living—manicured neighborhoods within a planned community, one small city hall and public library, three elementary schools, one middle school, and one high school. It's a place where kids' year-round sports games are held at one of two public parks, and you say "hello" to everyone you recognize at the grocery store. With only one Reform congregation, this town is where families build their lives, choosing it for its safety ranking and A-rated public schools. This is Parkland, Florida.

It used to be that when people asked me where I was from, I wouldn't even bother saying this small town's name. Located just south of Boca Raton and further west, bumping up against the Everglades, no one had heard of Parkland—that is, until February 14, 2018. A day known for love, flowers, and exchanging candy and sweet Valentines at school transformed into a hashtag: "#MSDstrong." This date marked a departure from children's and teens' innocence, as seventeen lives were taken and the words "semi-automatic," "AR-15," and "Code Red" became newly embedded in our vernacular.

That day marked my new understanding of the word "safety" and mistrust of its meaning; if you can't send your kids to school and expect them to be safe there, is anywhere safe?

February 14, 2018, also transformed my rabbinic and educational work. No longer was I the educator at a 250-family congregation; I had become a crisis counselor. Most of our synagogue's teens attended Marjory Stoneman Douglas High School and were at school that morning. While the senior rabbi and I were on our day off, we were inundated with a barrage of texts from a group of mothers in the community as the morning's horror unfolded in real time via social media and Snapchat videos.

After realizing what was happening in our town, I raced to get to work. What was normally a five-minute drive took over twenty minutes. Abandoned cars were scattered along the road, their doors left open as panicked parents rushed toward the high school in desperation. Code Red lockdowns were declared in all local public and private schools, including preschools.

When I arrived at the synagogue, ready to provide support and pastoral care to those in need, I asked our security guard to escort me inside, since I had to break the emergency protocol of no one being allowed to enter or leave the building. The senior rabbi arrived at about the same time, followed by our office staff, who stood still, holding their breath as they listened to their own teenage children tell them about hiding in classroom closets and bathrooms or behind barricaded doors—describing what they could or could not see and hear. Our synagogue's preschool teachers stayed locked in their classroom closets and restrooms with children ages four and younger, trying to keep them calm and entertained for several hours. My own children were just down the hall, hiding and confused.

Teens started to arrive at our door by foot, having escaped from the school and the shooter. They ran for their lives and arrived drenched in sweat to meet their parents and wait for other classmates. Those who could talk described what they saw and what they heard. Others remained silent in shock. By that evening, more teens had gathered and described their release after hours of hiding. It was painful to bear witness, hearing their stories of gunshots, blood-soaked hallways, stepping over dead bodies, and running for their lives. And how much more painful for those on the front lines, between only fourteen and eighteen years old.

Recounting the Days and Months After the Shooting: The Synagogue as a Sanctuary

The days and weeks following were a blur. As a barrage of funerals took place around town, we refocused our congregational priorities. It was no longer business as usual; we abandoned our regular programming to offer social, emotional, and spiritual care. Initially, we held an "emergency" healing service to gather our community and, later on, a community interfaith vigil.

The synagogue became a sanctuary—of mourning, reflection, and activism. Families came to us daily to seek refuge and togetherness. We set up a teen hangout space, had daily visits from therapy dogs, and had grief counselors on site for weeks following the tragedy. We started to offer meditation and yoga programs as well as hands-on service projects. With school closed, parents knew it was not healthy to keep their teens isolated, and so our halls were filled with families and students.

In moments like these, I tend to go into a focused "work mode," thinking systematically about what needs to be done and how best to do it. It is almost an out-of-body experience where I am able to set aside my own emotions and remain calm in order to get the work done. It is a bit surreal, moving through the steps and not allowing my feelings to overwhelm me.

Personal and Communal Healing Through Service and Ritual

My personal journey of healing intertwined with my professional role and challenged me in ways I could never have imagined, as I navigated my grief while supporting others. Every day brought a new challenge, whether it was helping to lead healing services or supporting the teens as they moved from shock and sadness to anger and then to action. The activism that arose in the aftermath became a powerful outlet for channeling our collective grief into a rallying cry against gun violence.

Providing rituals and services offered me a place to sit in my grief with local colleagues. The shared experiences we were facing—whether serving another Reform congregation or a church—bonded us as we navigated our new communal realities and responsibilities. These moments, whether in prayer, reflection, or activism, were profoundly healing for me. They reminded me of the strength found in community and the importance of standing together in times of crisis.

Yet, the importance of more personal self-care became increasingly evident as the months progressed. The blurred days became weeks and months of nonstop gear-switching between programs at the synagogue, pastoral counseling, and a new March for Our Lives movement, which needed adult support.

Activism: A Path Toward Communal Healing

The teens' questions started with "How could this happen?" and quickly evolved into "What can we do?" For many, the emotion translated to activism and leadership. Plans started for a youth group trip to Tallahassee to lobby the governor, and within five weeks, March for Our Lives set up nationwide marches. I worked alongside two synagogue teens who developed the March for our Lives Parkland chapter while witnessing two other youth groupers become prominent leaders in the larger movement. With a rabbinic colleague, we helped another student find her voice and speak on the main stage at March for Our Lives Los Angeles.

Our students wanted their voices to be heard. They fought for gun safety laws in Tallahassee and then in Washington. They wanted to take on the NRA and fight for increased background checks, longer waiting periods to purchase a gun, and a ban on assault rifles. They marched the urban streets of DC and the suburban streets of Parkland. They spoke at town halls and had lawmakers' cell phone numbers programmed into their phones. And they have been guests on more media outlets than I can count. So have I.

The Emotional Toll

At the same time as I stood beside and behind these teens, I counseled their families in my office and held them as they sobbed. While I had earned a master of social work degree prior to becoming a rabbi, I had not been prepared for this kind of work, dealing with communal trauma, while receiving my degrees in Jewish education and rabbinic ordination. And for this, I was so very angry at my graduate institution. In one day, my entire purpose at work changed. Colleagues offered support and love from afar. They sent our office staff meals and supplies to help make our youth lounge a comfortable space. But in the days and weeks following, some asked me to do things for them—find a teen to speak at a meeting or convention, review their lockdown and communication protocols, attend a conference myself to "share my story," and more. I was angry about this too. I needed my own shivah and *shloshim* period, and I felt that these rabbis should have recognized my pain.[1] Congregations and other organizations around the country sent us children's cards made in classrooms and art pieces, with expectations that they would be displayed, waiting not only for a "thank you" but also for photos and acknowledgments of receipt. This was a time when I tried to be fully present for those who needed me, instead of responding to these acts of kindness that had strings attached. It took me a long time to get past my resentment.

But some people and organizations showed up in creative ways I never imagined I needed. A close friend flew in to stay with me for two weeks and shadow me at work, in addition to cooking meals for my family and driving around my children. Other colleagues showed up at my synagogue to help create rituals and programs for my religious school teachers and students when I was too exhausted to think or plan. For this, I will forever be grateful.

Self-Care: My Most Hated Phrase That Year

During that year, many friends and colleagues would remind me, "Make sure you take care of yourself." I cognitively knew I needed to do this but found it difficult to carve out that time. I would enter my synagogue each morning as an empty vessel and allow others to fill me with their needs and stories. By the time I returned home at night, I was too exhausted to do much except try to empty myself back out to prepare for the next day.

The air in my community felt so heavy it was almost hard to breathe. I noticed this when I left town and traveled with the teens. When we were away, we could breathe, sleep, regroup, and recharge. One student I traveled with kept remarking about his exhaustion. The leaders of the program did not understand what he meant. Yes, he was tired from running around all day at an event and not sleeping as much at night, but it was more than that. It was the pure emotional exhaustion of trying to contain all of the emotions of the past year and function daily as the world expected a seventeen-year-old young man to do. I knew this feeling all too well. When I first left the community in May to attend a NFTY event at URJ Camp Coleman, I slept whenever I did not have to work. During the summer, while serving on faculty again at URJ Camp Coleman and then at Kutz Camp, I attended worship, cried a lot, and slept even more. I could barely discuss the shooting without tears welling up in my eyes. Distance gave me the chance to start to reflect on my own experiences. I realized how my body needed sleep and time to decompress. The summer also gave me the time to dwell in a happier space where the air was not enveloped in grief and anger. However, it felt peculiar being surrounded by joy, yet feeling so emotionally detached. It provided a much-needed respite to recharge and restore some balance.

Moving Forward Grounded in Jewish Values

In the years following the shooting, I became a resident expert for the Reform Movement on teen crisis, communal trauma, and acts of gun violence. I toured professional conferences to speak about how to prepare for the worst and the experience of getting sent in to help in the aftermath of painful situations. The time that has passed has created a distance that allows me to share in raw, vulnerable ways while still being able to speak without choking on my words. It has been cathartic in some ways, but often it reopens tender wounds.

The shooting of February 14, 2018, will forever be part of the psyche of my community. We have risen from the pain, but there are indelible marks on all of us. There are constant reminders of the lives lost everywhere you turn, from memorials outside the high school and in neighborhoods to crimson ribbons printed on the jersey of every child playing for city-sponsored sports teams. Indeed, the sponsors emblazoned on the backs of children's sports jerseys are often the nonprofits started by Parkland parents in memory of their dead children. The increased police presence is always noticed, and every school practices monthly lockdown drills. Mental health and bullying issues are quickly addressed when they bubble up in public schools.

The aftermath of the tragedy has brought a lot of good. Beautiful nonprofits support school safety and teen programming. Children now have a half-day at school on February 14 each year, and it is always framed as a day of service and love. Anniversary gatherings continue in public communal settings, drawing an interfaith community for prayer.

This hometown tragedy of Parkland tested our capacity for resilience and our ability to make sense of the world. Yet, through the lens of social action and *tikkun olam*, the teens and families found a pathway through the trauma. Our response—rooted in activism, community support, and personal healing—illustrates the transformative power of Judaism to guide us through the darkest of times. This communal response revealed our personal strength, the power of community, and the unyielding hope for a better future. In remembering the lives lost and the resilience gained, we remain a community transformed and scarred, moving forward with a commitment to heal ourselves, to fix broken political systems desperately in need of repair, and to advocate for change to make the world a more compassionate and safer place for all. The teens led the charge; it is up to us to support them.

And for me, I learned the value of community and friendship. I will forever remember those who stepped up to support me—Melissa—so that I—Rabbi Stollman—could be present for others. But most importantly, I learned that I have far more tenacity than I ever realized and that self-care is vital. Just as the safety instructions on airplanes suggest, we need to place our oxygen masks on ourselves before helping others. I learned the importance of caring for myself, of taking time to mourn and rest.

The City of Parkland has been added to a list containing the names of towns like Sandy Hook and Columbine; it will be remembered for the tragedy that took the lives of teenagers. But I will remember the strength, the resilience, and the compassion found among neighbors, friends, and strangers. I will remember the inner strength I discovered and will draw upon it often.

NOTE
1. Shivah is the seven-day period of intense mourning following burial. *Sh'loshim* is the thirty-day period of less intense mourning customs following burial.

25

From Brokenness to Blessing

Serving as a Chaplain in Pittsburgh
After the Tree of Life Massacre

RABBI SHIRA STERN, DMIN, BCC

As a chaplain in an acute-care health-care hospital, I often visited with patients who had not requested pastoral care, but who were part of my unit responsibilities. Sometimes the patients were open to talking; sometimes they were in too much pain or discomfort and asked that I return later. And once in a while, I entered a room and was faced with anger, hostility, and abusive language—a tsunami of frustration. I didn't take it personally: I was simply the safest person on whom that patient could unload their extreme emotional and spiritual angst.

I had two responses. The first was to apologize for intruding and then retreat. The second was to allow them to vent, without interruption or judgment, in the hope that once the fury had dissipated, they might want to talk. Regardless of which path I chose, those were difficult encounters.

Then Biblical Esau spoke to me:

> Just as Isaac finished blessing Jacob, at the very moment that Jacob was in the act of leaving his father Isaac's presence, his brother Esau came in from his hunt.
>
> He too made tasty dishes that he brought to his father and he said to his father, "Let my father get ready to eat of his son's game, so that you can give me your heartfelt blessing."
>
> But his father Isaac said to him, "Who are you?" So he replied, "I am your son, your first-born, Esau!"
>
> Isaac now began to shudder—a shuddering exceedingly great—and he said, "Who then hunted game and brought [it] to me and I ate of it all before you came? I blessed him—and blessed he will remain!"
>
> When Esau heard his father's words, he broke into an exceedingly loud and bitter howl and said to his father, "Bless me! Me too, Father!

> But he said, "Your brother came with deceit and took away your blessing!"
>
> He replied, "Is he not named Jacob? Twice now he has cheated me—he took my birthright and now, look, he has taken my blessing!" And he added, "Did you not reserve a blessing for me?"
>
> Isaac responded by saying to Esau, "Look—I have appointed him your master, and given him all his kin to be his servants, and have supported him with grain and new wine; come, now, what am I to do, my son?"
>
> "Do you have but one blessing, Father?" said Esau to his father. "Bless me! Me too, Father!" And Esau cried out and wept." (Genesis 27:30–38)

Suddenly, I heard in my patient's anger the echo of the son whose birthright and blessing had been stolen from him. It was a cry that came from the depths of his being. *Isn't there a blessing for me too? Didn't God reserve some special blessing that could help me in this awful situation? God, do You really only have one blessing to give?* When faced with trauma, we often ask ourselves, "Are all the blessings taken? Where can I find *my* blessing?"

This Biblical passage has defined my disaster and health-care chaplaincy ever since. In order to listen to the suffering of my patients, allowing them their "sacred screaming,"[1] I first have to figure out what they are feeling and what their internal and external resources are. What will they need to turn the intense negative energy into something that will bring them closer to healing? What can I, as a chaplain, do to alleviate some of that pain? What will I say, or sing, or bring them?

I thought of all these things in the late morning of October 27, 2018. I received a call asking me to deploy immediately to Pittsburgh with the Red Cross, in response to the massacre that had just occurred at Tree of Life synagogue, a building housing three separate minyanim (prayer communities). Eleven congregants had died, more were wounded, and the perpetrator was being treated at an area hospital. At this juncture, no one knew why or how this happened. I sat on my couch, stunned and shattered to my core.

As a disaster spiritual care manager for the Red Cross, and at that point having been part of the organization for almost eighteen years, I had learned that every disaster is different, even if they look the same. Yet, in every situation, each volunteer has the responsibility to care for clients, fellow staff, and volunteers. Most importantly, we are in this for the long haul, so we must take care of ourselves.

Having deployed to Ground Zero for months after 9/11, to the Boston Marathon bombing, and to several dozen major weather-related disasters, I thought I was ready for the task at hand. I would make sure I debriefed every evening with my team; I would be in regular contact with friends and family; I would seek out and be well supported by the local Red Cross chapter.

And yet, three months later, when the Jewish Bluegrass group Nefesh Mountain came to our shul for a concert and played their tribute to Tree of Life, I sat in the front of the sanctuary in a puddle of tears I could not control. I was transported back to the intense state of mourning I found when I arrived in Pittsburgh. I remembered standing with neighbors on Squirrel Hill at the makeshift memorials as they remembered their friends. I recalled visiting with families who had lost loved ones, whose private sadness had become public events. I was once again visiting area synagogues, instructing religious school teachers about how to broach the topic of trauma with their students and communities and best allow them to process their feelings of vulnerability.

Somewhere during that first deployment to Pittsburgh, I began to see the blessings emerging amid the trauma.

I remember sitting with the debriefing circle of the *chevrah kadisha*, the amazing team of volunteers who had gently washed the mangled bodies and prepared them for burial. We listened for two and a half hours as both experienced and brand-new members slowly allowed themselves to share their pain, bearing witness to the horror. The group was a mix of men and women from every stage of life and from many different spiritual communities. For some, this was a difficult but familiar responsibility; for others, it was the first time they had ever completed the ritual of *tohorah*.[2] But they all had one thing in common: They felt a calling to mitigate the damage by doing their extraordinary sacred work. Ideological differences did not matter. They were one group who understood their shared mission. Claiming that feeling was, in itself, a blessing.

When you can regroup, you can survive: That is the key to moving from tragedy to resilience.

After my first trip, I returned to Pittsburgh four more times to work with youth groups and Jewish communal leaders and to attend the first memorial service. Five years later, that deployment continues to impact my life not only because of what I saw, but because of the power of hope and connection in everyone around me. Within hours of the initial event, the shock and grief were transformed into action by both the Jewish community and the greater Pittsburgh community, who were present for one another. At the shivahs I attended, I often saw members of other grieving families. At every Shabbat or weekday service, there were extended families who had flown in or driven across the country to show everyone affected that they were not alone. I saw complete strangers, many of whom were not Jewish, offer solace, dedicate memorials, and create banners intended to strengthen the Squirrel Hill community. Amid the relived pain, both physical and psychological, were those moments of great beauty. They created harmony to offset the anguish, committing themselves to finding joy in life despite it all, and many formed new lifelong friendships.

In the summer of 2023, I spent time with the same families as they attended the three-month-long trial of the shooter. He continued to feel no remorse for what he had done. For many of the survivors, this intransigence was infuriating. Some worked out their anger by marching up and down the halls; others quietly went to another place within themselves to protect the wounds that would always exist. It was clear that no adjudication or sentence would bring back their loved ones; those emotional scars were permanent.

But a group of Jewish social workers, psychologists, and Jewish chaplains—myself included—tried to mitigate a little of that pain by providing rotating support to the families each day of the trial. Sometimes we sat with them in the actual courtroom, though doing so meant having to show no emotion whatsoever in response to the testimony until we were outside in the adjacent corridors. At other times, we sat in the unoccupied courtroom one floor above, with a live feed on TV providing a continual combination of infuriating or tedious, methodical arguments, listening to the families react to the drama unfolding in real time. Survivors were given a choice to testify, thus ensuring that *their* story was part of the evidence the judge and jury would take into account when they decided on the verdict and the sentence. Repeatedly, I heard people say that although they had their own narratives, despite the fact that the community had provided regular support groups to the families, no one had a complete picture of the events that unfolded that day until they heard the individual accounts during the proceedings.

No one can fully prepare themselves for what happens in life, but our job as spiritual care providers is to offer these four components of basic chaplaincy:

1. Recognize that each person is a living human document.[3]
2. Walk with the person in their suffering.
3. Help them to articulate their truth.
4. Help them to articulate their prayer.

My goal is to help others wrest blessing from brokenness, even if that blessing is not the blessing they anticipated. Every single person—like a Torah—deserves our focus; every person deserves our respect; every person deserves to be treated with dignity and be heard, even when what they share is painful. By affirming a person's story, by sitting with them in their grief, we can help that individual, family, or community find a new blessing to comfort them and then to sustain them. The goal is to clear a path toward resiliency.

The dictionary defines resilience as "power or ability to return to the original form, position, etc., after being bent, compressed, or stretched."[4] However, human resilience, once bent or compressed or stretched, does not mean that we can go back to what we were before. We always carry the scars, both internal and external, when life is upended. Resilience lies not in some achievable goal, but in being able to pick oneself up when it is the hardest thing in the world to do, over and over and over again. In tiny steps. In small increments. And some-times, it also lies in accepting that after taking one small step forward, one can go two steps backward and not lose everything.

Accessing the tools to find our own resilience in the face of trauma is the key to our survival and healing. The question is: How do we harness both our inner and external resources? What tools can we use to help us become more resilient? Can we find a way after suffering from trauma to build on past experiences so that we return to a place of healing and equilibrium? What can we glean from others that will inform *our* behavior so that we might survive difficult situations more easily?

My answer to that requires accessing the world of the spirit.

First, I need to know the context: What happened, to whom did it happen, and what means does the person have to pull themselves back from despair? I start with a prayer, because the ritual of saying it helps me focus, like putting on sneakers to work out, or wearing a helmet to bike ride, or lighting a *yahrzeit* candle to commemorate a loved one's death. It is usually short: "God—just help me do this," or maybe "Help me find the right words."

After the focusing prayer, I hum to myself the following piece of liturgy; I find that the reverberations in my throat from chanting help me concentrate more efficiently.

> *Kol han'shamah t'haleil Yah. Hal'luyah!*
> My whole soul praises God. Hallelujah!

In this song, the word for soul, *n'shamah*, also means "breath." My very breath praises God. My whole being praises You. Like a mantra, I'll repeat the line several times until, even when I'm feeling really down, I begin to believe it myself. *Kol han'shamah t'haleil Yah, Hal'luyah.*

I then take the word *N'ShaMaH* and begin a simple four-part checklist that will force me to focus on the details of the encounter. It becomes a trigger for spiritual situational awareness.

Name That Emotion: What am I feeling?[5]

Abandonment	Anticipation	Courage
Isolation	Hope	Gratitude
Joy	Love	Sadness
Depression	Despair	Forgiveness

Show the Support: What keeps me going?

My internal resources	strong/weak	present/not present
Family resources	strong/weak	present/not present
Friend resources	strong/weak	present/not present
Community resources	strong/weak	present/not present

Make It Happen: Do something:

Life review	Spontaneous prayer	*Vidui*[6]
Mi Shebeirach[7]	Social joining	Therapeutic presence

Heighten the Healing:
Music/scent/quiet/light

My goal is to enable others to find their own blessings and use them as building blocks for a new life. Viktor Frankl said, "Man is *not* fully conditioned and determined but rather determines himself whether he gives into conditions or stands up to them."[8] I know it isn't easy to stand up to difficult conditions, tragedy, or trauma. Most of us have felt like we are hanging on to this life by a thread, whether it's for a moment or some protracted time. Resilience is not the constant bright light that shines our way ahead, but is instead getting up each day to rekindle the tiny flame. Rabbi Steven Kushner points out that the original *ner tamid*, the "eternal light," wasn't eternal at all; it required the Israelites to renew the oil and the wick each and every day.[9] The same thing is required of our own light. Day after day, whether we anticipate great joy or are unaware of what is about to happen, we still wake up and reignite the flame.

Sometimes, that is about all the energy we can muster. Sometimes, it's the starting point for a great move forward—the beginning of fighting for and finding one's own blessing.

When Jacob steals the blessing from Esau, the intensity of Esau's pain is palpable. The twin who is a "hunter" rather than a "gatherer," who is seen as the strong, silent type rather than the more sensitive personality, reveals his suffering and his vulnerability. But that is not where the story ends. In fact, Isaac *does* have another blessing for Esau, though not the one Esau expected or thought he deserved. When Esau cries out, "Have you but one blessing, Father? Bless me too, Father!" Isaac answers, "Lo, among the fat places of the earth shall your dwelling be, and with heaven's dew from above. By your sword shall you serve. But when you move away, you shall break his yoke off your neck" (Genesis 27:39–40).

For twenty years, the brothers neither see nor contact one another. Then Jacob comes back to see if he can reconcile with Esau. To prepare for the encounter, Jacob divides his family and his worldly possessions, in case Esau still has murder on his mind. Overnight, Jacob "wrestles with the angel of destiny and inner conflict and says, 'I will not let you go until you bless me.' That is how he rescues hope from catastrophe—as Jews have always done. Their darkest nights have always been preludes to their most creative dawns."[10]

For surviving families in Pittsburgh, for those of us for whom the attack on Tree of Life was a sea change in the way we saw the world, finding blessing in the aftermath almost feels disloyal. How can we possibly see anything good emerge from this tragedy? Should we preserve the memory of that day just as it was, or should we acknowledge the fragile healing that time and distance have allowed to grow? Carole Zawatsky, chief executive of Tree of Life, was asked about the anticipated new building that will house a new sanctuary, a museum about antisemitism, and an education center "where difficult questions can be debated and discussed." She said, "It is more a space that honors and explores these complicated issues."[11] If we are to move forward from this abyss, we have to be willing to have these disparate feelings coexisting within us. Only in acknowledging the struggle can we make meaning from it.

That is what we try to offer—a way to find blessing that will enable us to continue after a cataclysmic loss. It reminds us that when we bring this healing to ourselves and others, we partner with God.

NOTES
1. Lori Lefkovitz and Rona Shapiro, "Ritualwell.Org—Loading the Virtual Canon, or: The Politics and Aesthetics of Jewish Women's Spirituality," *Nashim: A Journal of Jewish Women's Studies & Gender Issues*, no. 9 (Spring 2005): 101–25, http://www.jstor.org/stable/40326620.
2. The ritual of washing a body three times before wrapping it in a shroud.
3. This term was coined by Anton T. Boisen, who is understood to be the founder of the clinical pastoral education movement. Boisen "firmly believed that a firsthand study of human experience—what he called a reading of the 'living human documents'—was a necessary supplement to classroom training." See Glenn H. Asquith, "Anton T. Boisen and the Study of 'Living Human Documents,'" *Journal of Presbyterian History (1962–1985)* 60, no. 3 (1982): 244–65, http://www.jstor.org/stable/23328440.
4. See "Resilience," in *Dictionary.Com*, accessed June 14, 2024, https://www.dictionary.com/browse/resilience.
5. Thanks to Rabbi Elizabeth Rolle for this terminology.
6. The *Vidui* is the confessional prayer said at the end of life and on Yom Kippur.
7. The *Mi Shebeirach* is the prayer for healing of body and spirit.
8. Viktor E. Frankl, *Man's Search for Meaning: An Introduction to Logotherapy*, 4th ed. (Beacon Press, 1992), 133.

9. Steven Kushner, "Quest for Fire" (Temple Ner Tamid, March 2009), https://images.shulcloud.com/13511/uploads/Documents/Kushner/QuestForFire.pdf.

10. Rabbi Jonathan Sacks, "Jacob's Destiny, Israel's Name," in *Covenant & Conversation: A Weekly Reading of the Jewish Bible, Genesis: The Book of Beginnings* (Maggid Books & The Orthodox Union, 2009), 240.

11. Campbell Robertson, "Tree of Life Synagogue to Break Ground on New Sanctuary, and New Mission," *New York Times*, June 22, 2024, https://www.nytimes.com/2024/06/22/us/tree-of-life-groundbreaking.html.

PART FIVE

Trauma from Natural Disasters and Pandemics

26

Floods, Winds, and Wheels
Lessons from Hurricane Katrina

Rabbi Robert H. Loewy

THE END OF AUGUST 2005 presented two traumatic challenges indelibly etched in my memory: one solely personal, the second both personal and communal.

On Monday evening, August 22, my wife, Lynn, our daughter Sara, and I checked into a hotel in Austin, Texas, about to commence Sara's freshman year at the University of Texas. The next morning, we discovered our rear car window smashed and most of Sara's possessions stolen. First came incredulity, then tears. We knew that some items were easily replaced while others were not. Forced to be resilient, we quickly conceived a plan to recoup what we could, repair the car, deal with the insurance company, and enable Sara to move into her residence.

On August 24, we bid our daughter farewell as she began her college career, and we headed home to Metairie, Louisiana, a suburb of New Orleans. We were all a bit shaken, but satisfied at having effectively addressed the challenge. I celebrated my fifty-fifth birthday on August 25, cognizant of portentous words that still prompt anxiety and occasional action since I first became rabbi of Congregation Gates of Prayer in 1984: "There's a storm in the Gulf."

Hurricanes, at least, provide warning. We had evacuated numerous times before 2005, including the previous year over Rosh HaShanah for Hurricane Ivan. On some occasions the flight was for naught as the storms made landfall far from our home, but we can never be sure where they will go. And so we were vigilant, preparing just in case with personal and congregational checklists developed from experience. On August 26, the storm was dangerously large, predicted to be severe, with Greater New Orleans (NOLA) in the center of the "cone of uncertainty."

With the storm track unchanged and the Jewish value of *pikuach nefesh*—preservation of life—paramount, my family (Lynn, younger daughter, Mica, and dog, Sushi) and the congregation decided it was time to evacuate. So, on the morning of August 27, the Temple staff and I wrapped the Torahs in plastic and moved them to the fifth floor of a local office building. Then my family and I packed one of our cars to flee. The usual five-and-a-half-hour drive to Houston took ten hours with evacuation traffic. We arrived in Houston at 3:00 a.m. on August 28; from there we would anxiously watch and wait, uncertain as to how this dangerous storm might impact our lives.

Hurricane Katrina struck Greater New Orleans in the early morning of Monday, August 29, with 140 mph winds and heavy rain, but initial reports were that NOLA had mostly been spared. That evening, I gathered many other Houston evacuees for a service held at Congregation Emanu El, giving thanks for once again dodging a bullet. I recall comforting the mother of a bride-to-be that all would be well. Later that night began the reports of levee breaches in New Orleans, with water cascading into homes and businesses. Not as severe, but similarly destructive, the drainage system that pumps water from the streets in Metairie also failed.

At least 80 percent of the City of New Orleans came under water by August 31, ultimately resulting in 1,833 fatalities and $108 billion in damages.[1] Metairie suffered comparatively minor flooding but still sustained major damage, since water stayed in buildings for days. Our home—filled with eighteen inches of water—sustained $120,000 in losses; the synagogue's losses were well over a million dollars; approximately 75 percent of my congregants had enough damage necessitating they live elsewhere or in FEMA trailers.

We were not the first to experience a natural disaster, but Katrina was unique in a variety of ways. An entire city and metropolitan area were impacted, as people from all levels of the socioeconomic ladder suffered. Adding to the misery was the fact that much of the damage was directly related not just to the storm but to human failures. Constant coverage by cable news networks and images shared on nascent social media regularly featured homeless and destitute people seeking refuge at the Superdome or the Convention Center, neither of which were equipped as shelters. Jewish media shared pictures of Torah scrolls being rescued, only later to be buried, having been soaked and damaged beyond repair. Sadly, this was just the first of many such storms, now understood to be related to climate change, that dominate the headlines annually.

Looking back, I realize that Katrina and its aftermath were the most challenging and meaningful period of my rabbinate. The gravity of the situation was apparent by August 31; the future, though, remained unclear. I was devastated to see the destruction and its impact upon so many. Personally, I was scared and uncertain, my usual calm replaced by nervousness and angst. Could our home be renovated? Would I have a job, with congregants scattered across the country? Would they return? Would they be able to meet their financial obligations to the synagogue? Could the congregation pay my salary? Where would our youngest daughter go to school? Would my wife have her job? The uncertainty was initially paralyzing. While my head knew that eventually all would be well, I was overwhelmed at the present challenges. Then the personal and professional adrenaline kicked in.

Dealing with our family situation was relatively straightforward. We rented an apartment in Houston and enrolled Mica in the Jewish day school that opened its doors to the NOLA evacuees. Authorities prohibited us from returning home for almost two weeks; once I was allowed to return for a few hours, I was able to retrieve some essential belongings and begin the process of flood cleanup and restoration. Our downstairs was a disaster zone, but fortunately the second floor was untouched. I was also able to recover two of our cars, which we had parked at a nearby garage.

Then I went to the synagogue and walked through the building with my flashlight. The center of our synagogue sanctuary was literally a sunken area that we referred to as "the well"; now, water reflecting off my beam overflowed the well and filled the sanctuary. I loaded my car with boxes of *machzorim* (High Holy Day prayer books) to bring to Houston. With Rosh HaShanah approaching in October, I imagined holding services but knew they would not be in Metairie. Most congregants had evacuated to Houston and Baton Rouge, others to Atlanta, Memphis, and numerous other points on the globe. I was blessed with a dedicated administrator and strong lay leaders who focused on physical reconstruction, while my cantorial soloist and I concentrated on rebuilding the spiritual congregation. It started to sink in that we were not the first Jewish community to be displaced by forces beyond our control, nor would we be the last. My role was to look to the future.

The first challenge was to locate the members. Not everyone had email at the time, and cell phones from NOLA were inoperable. Frantically I began the process of recreating our temple's roster, which ultimately took over a year to complete. I was in Super Rabbi mode, glued to my phone or computer for hours, attempting to make contact and trying to reimagine how I could continue to serve—pastorally, spiritually, and practically.

Reestablishing a sense of community was the first step. During the first month after the storm, we gathered in Houston and Baton Rouge for services and group meals. In cooperation with my colleague Rabbi Andy Busch of Touro Synagogue and with the support of the Union for Reform Judaism (URJ), we rented space to hold Rosh HaShanah and Yom Kippur services for those who were dispersed to Houston and Baton Rouge. (Yes, I certainly used that concept of being in the diaspora in my communications. Greater New Orleans may not be *Eretz Yisrael* [the Land of Israel], but it was our homeland.)

As I served my congregants' needs, I realized that they were simultaneously addressing my own. Feeling connection to community and experiencing something normal like High Holy Day services brought healing to us all.

That Rosh HaShanah evening—speaking to those who had evacuated from New Orleans, along with additional families from Beaumont, Texas, who had fled from Hurricane Rita—I attempted to respond to the question "Where is God?" I turned to I Kings 19:11–12, which describes how the prophet Elijah was forced to take refuge from those who wished to kill him. He arrived at Mount Sinai and entered a cave, where he spent the night. God called to him to come out of the cave and stand on the mountain. Then, "the Eternal passed by. There was a great and mighty wind, splitting mountains and shattering rocks by the power of the Eternal, but God was not in the wind. After the wind—an earthquake, but God was not in the earthquake. After the earthquake—fire, but God was not in the fire." Then I added, "After the fire—torrential rains and floods, but God was not in the waters," after which I returned to the Biblical text. "And after the waters, a soft, murmuring sound, a still, small voice."

I explained the text by saying, "My friends, God is not in the hurricanes. Katrina and Rita were not acts of God, but simply of nature, part of the forces in our world, which are simply random. God did not sit around and say, 'Last year was Florida's turn, I think this year it is finally time for New Orleans and Beaumont. After all, they are overdue.' I just don't believe God works in that fashion. God is that still, small voice that spoke to us when we lost faith and courage. God is the presence that reminds us there will be tomorrow and we will have the strength to face it. God provides us with a path to share our fears and know that we are never alone." Though addressing the community, I was speaking to myself as well.

God was also in the countless acts of kindness that so many of us experienced in the aftermath of the storm. It started with the support of family, particularly our parents and adult children, Karen Loewy with her husband, Rabbi David Widzer, and our son, David. For the first time in my life and for most of my congregants, we found ourselves in real need. Normally *tzedakah* was something we gave, not received. A key concept I taught my congregants through written and oral communication—and by personal example—was the idea that "*tzedakah* is a wheel," based upon the Babylonian Talmud teaching found in *Shabbat* 151b: "Rabbi Chiya advised his wife, 'When a poor person comes to the door, be quick to give them food so that the same may be done to your children.' She exclaimed, 'You are cursing our children [with the suggestion that they may become beggars].' But Rabbi Chiya replied, 'There is a wheel that revolves in this world.'"

The wheel had turned. We who were displaced from our homes, facing steep unanticipated financial challenges, needed to be open to receiving FEMA assistance, Red Cross support, and grants available from the local Jewish Family Service. This included me and my family, and I availed myself of *tzedakah* out of need and to role-model for others.

Following an appeal that I made on RAVKAV, the Reform rabbinic listserv, my Rabbi's Discretionary Fund swelled, and we were inundated with gift cards. Acts of *g'milut chasadim* (loving-kindness) enabled me to distribute significant amounts of financial assistance directly to hundreds of people. Many would not accept checks but found gift cards easier to receive.

In the middle of October, I returned to my home and synagogue, while my family remained safe in Houston. I lived on the second floor of my house with a mini refrigerator, toaster oven, and microwave, as if I were a college student. The downstairs was bare, concrete and studs. The synagogue had a similar décor—concrete floors, walls ripped out to the studs, with folding chairs and tables serving as office furniture. Floodwaters and winds left destruction and debris everywhere. Trash, ruined appliances, furniture, carpeting—the remnants of homes and lives—were piled high on every street. All around me was dust and grime. I felt a compulsion to keep washing my hands, even when unnecessary; this feeling stayed with me for years.

Still, it felt good to be back, knowing we were on the path to rebuilding our homes, congregation, and community. Most of the participants in the limited activities we offered were those whose homes had been spared; the remainder were living either in FEMA trailers, in rental properties, or with friends.

Shabbat services became a time to come together for something familiar, though we were always cognizant of the trauma we had endured. My *divrei Torah* (words of Torah, sermons) offered themes of hope, renewal, and comfort—themes I needed to hear about as much as my congregants. Our worship custom of sharing personal examples of gratitude, linked to the *Hodaah* (Thanksgiving) prayer, became basic and cathartic: "I am thankful for having electricity." "We have sheetrock." "Internet and cable have been restored."

During those first few months, the synagogue provided Shabbat dinners each week, as most of us had no kitchens. We also developed programs to deal with practical and emotional needs. We even brought in a comedian, scholars, and music programs to lift our spirits. Over time, our numbers grew as we adjusted to the "new normal." For me and all who experienced Katrina directly, time is measured "BK" and "AK"—before and after Katrina.

Pirkei Avot 1:14 served to frame my personal and our communal response: "If I am not for myself, who will be?" First, we had to rebuild our own homes and congregation. With the help of the local Federation, the URJ, and numerous other organizations and individuals, we were able to do so. On a personal level, I also realized that after a long period of trying to be Super Rabbi, I needed to take breaks to rest, relax, and refresh. I could take off my "Super Rabbi cape" to exercise, watch sports, or work on something other than recovery efforts; I was then better able to confront the tasks at hand.

Pirkei Avot 1:14 continues, "But if I am only for myself, who am I? And if not now, when?" Clearly our "now" was a time for action. We were blessed with support to rebuild. The same could not be said for people living in poorer neighborhoods, particularly within the Black community. It was fulfilling to be part of groups that physically helped strangers empty their homes of debris. I was proud to be the conduit of Jewish funds to churches, HBCUs, and a variety of other institutions in Greater New Orleans. Many Jews led in rebuilding the educational system, and my synagogue actively supported the creation of a homeless shelter for women and children located in the devastated Ninth Ward.

Now—decades after Katrina—my anxiety level still rises at the beginning of every hurricane season and does not decrease until it ends. I've evacuated many times since 2005 but have been relatively unscathed, knowing storms and fires have devastated others. The *tzedakah* wheel has turned, and we are once again able to be donors. While I recognize that each natural disaster is different, it is gratifying to support colleagues with funds and counsel based on my experience as they confront their unique challenges.

The first major trauma I ever dealt with was the loss of a child; that trauma propelled me to write an article to help rabbis who might face the same loss.[2] At that time, I could not have imagined twenty years later I would face anything even comparably challenging. A major difference was that with Katrina, I was one of thousands to endure this ordeal. One never fully recovers from a real trauma, but we can learn to use it to help ourselves and others deal with the next storm—literal or figurative—that comes our way.

(And by the way—my family now avoids leaving luggage in our car overnight in hotel parking lots.)

Notes

1. Jeffrey Medlin et al., "Extremely Powerful Hurricane Katrina Leaves a Historic Mark on the Northern Gulf Coast: A Killer Hurricane Our Country Will Never Forget," National Weather Service, updated September 2022, https://www.weather.gov/mob/katrina.
2. Robert H. Loewy, "A Rabbi Confronts Miscarriage, Stillbirth, and Infant Death," *Journal of Reform Judaism* 35, no. 2 (Spring 1988), 1–6.

27

The Rising Floodwaters
Surviving Hurricane Harvey

RABBI ADRIENNE P. SCOTT

PREPARING for a major flood and its aftermath was not part of any course I took at Hebrew Union College–Jewish Institute of Religion. However, when I began my service as a rabbi at Congregation Beth Israel in Houston, Texas, in June 2005, hurricanes became a part of our regular fall planning schedule. When these events caused power to go out, our clergy team relocated to plan for services in conference rooms of apartment buildings, coffee shops, or wherever else we could find power and a table large enough to fit us. In the early 2000s, I knew nothing of Zoom or Teams. We planned for alternative locations for services and bet mitzvah ceremonies and even joined congregations in other cities around the state to observe *S'lichot* and Rosh HaShanah.

Houston became a significant absorption center when Hurricane Katrina barreled through New Orleans in the late summer of 2005. Our clergy team and lay leadership, in conjunction with the Jewish Federation of Greater Houston, connected families who had lost touch with one another. We hosted social events for children so that parents would have time to handle work matters. It was hectic, overwhelming, and rewarding all at the same time. When Hurricane Rita struck shortly after Katrina in 2005, I, like many Houstonians, spent fifteen hours in the car with my family in an effort to reach Dallas, Texas—normally a four-hour trip.

In 2008, we experienced firsthand the intensity of Hurricane Ike. Most homes within the Houston area were without power for nearly two weeks. As a new mother, I remember taking my daughter in her car seat to meet congregants and provide pastoral care for those dealing with significant loss. Life didn't stop simply because of a hurricane. The funerals, hospital visits, and phone calls kept coming. It was a balance of patience, compassion, and care like no other time. I couldn't stop, pause, or reflect on any other needs. I was in full survival mode—taking it day by day, and sometimes hour by hour—without any day care. Slowly, life returned to a new normal, and I incorporated my experience of trauma as I continued to develop my rabbinate. That is, until 2017, when Hurricane Harvey came to Houston.

By this time, our community had become more adept at handling these natural disasters. Floods in 2015 and 2016 were like an appetizer for Harvey's main course. As a congregation, we stayed updated on the news reports of the impending storm. We safeguarded our temple and ensured that our Torah scrolls were safe. Because of the anticipated grim forecast, we canceled Shabbat services. However, as a clergy team, we came together to create a *Havdalah* video that we posted to Facebook. This was somewhat revolutionary in 2017. We initially thought that the storm may have missed us, but come Motza-ei Shabbat on Saturday night, the rains came and didn't stop for hours and hours. Floodwaters rose quickly and furiously throughout the city. Lawns became pools. Streets became rivers. Even homes not in the floodplain became inundated with several feet of water. Since buildings have no basements, floodwaters in Houston have nowhere else to go, and the city was quickly overwhelmed. We were living through a one-hundred-year flood of Biblical proportions—without Noah or any ark to save us. My in-laws had to evacuate as they became inundated, and even crossing the street was dangerous with the floodwaters rapidly rising.

It was difficult for me to even get to the temple, a trip that normally takes ten minutes. There were many road closures and ongoing flooding, but as soon as we could, the clergy, senior staff, and lay leaders went to our main sanctuary. Nearly half of the room was filled with water; we needed to begin the remediation process immediately. With rainboots and masks, we began removing prayer books and carefully taking stock of the damage. Our feet sloshed with the sound of the water. It was disheartening. Congregation Beth Israel is near Brays Bayou, an open reservoir that should have been able to hold and retain the water. Due to the intense nature of the hurricane, not even the bayou could sustain the amount and the speed of the rising water. It overflowed onto the streets and surrounding homes, leaving streets completely covered for days after the hurricane initially made landfall.

We quickly set up a crisis center in our offices. We divided our membership directory based on zip codes and began assessing the damage. Hundreds of our congregants and thousands in our city were impacted by the storm. Donations began to pour in rapidly from congregants, colleagues, and friends from across the country. Their *chesed* was beyond kind and generous at a time when our congregation needed it the most. As we are taught, *kol Yisrael areivim zeh bazeh* (Babylonian Talmud, *Sh'vuot* 39a)—each person is responsible for another—and we were living proof of this principle and teaching. To this day, I am reminded of this by the notes and cards I received and still have in my office, which provided me with comfort and a sense of gratitude.

Experiencing a flood means living with a natural disaster for many days and weeks. The intense aroma of warped wood, the sight of heaps of household trash, and the smell of mildew are something I can still recall. Finding time for self-care was challenging, as I was unable to enjoy my regular running route. The piles of waste were enormous and took up entire front lawns, sidewalks, and other passageways. Addresses were hard to find because the house numbers were blocked by layers of garbage. I couldn't even park on the street in front of congregants' houses because there was no other place for the debris to go.

The pastoral work was all-consuming. As a rabbi, I was fully present, on the front lines, and each day woke up to new challenges that needed to be triaged. I helped displaced families with their personal needs, obtained school supplies, and located cleaning equipment. I was like a zombie on autopilot, called to help others who had been affected, to remove clothing and other damaged items, and to find resources and help. The calls from across the country from rabbinic colleagues were a gesture that was so appreciated and desperately needed. This bittersweet reality of knowing how much work needed to be done and that so many others were helping was a comfort to me and so many other leaders in our community.

Throughout this entire period, our community came together. With tears and feelings of profound loss for personal heirlooms, family homes, and a rapidly changing community, we truly felt like we had been wandering through the desert. Like the Biblical Nachshon ben Ammi-nadab, who our Rabbinic commentators note was the first to enter the waters of the Sea of Reeds before it began to part, each member of our community needed to act and rebuild. With faith in our first steps from the water onto dry land, we focused on our mental health and provided for every member of our sacred community. The days were unending and often unforgiving. We quickly learned to manage countless data-bases with ever-changing information on our congregants and their new addresses. We hosted community dinners where we offered attend-ees cleaning supplies and other food items to help get them through the initial challenges. Our lay leaders gave their time to help make phone calls, provide food for the staff, and maintain optimism when hope and comfort were scarce. Each day blurred together, but we did our best to provide for others while maintaining our own well-being.

One of the biggest challenges was that schools remained out of ses-sion. Parents couldn't care for their children and also focus on the reme-diation of their homes. Our temple was deeply committed to the Jewish value of welcoming guests, *hachnasat orchim*. Alongside other congre-gations and community organizations, we came together to offer day camps and other invaluable programs to support families. We even had the space and ability to host a local Jewish day school that also suffered significant damage. Our social hall was transformed into school rooms, akin to a *beit midrash* (house of study) of old. Our sacred worship spaces were used by other congregations to observe bet mitzvah. We were grateful for the opportunity to make sure that nothing had to be further postponed or canceled, as we are taught not to delay joy.

The first Shabbat service we held at Congregation Beth Israel the week after the storm was tearful and challenging. Nearly everyone who attended had experienced flooding in some capacity, large or small. It was a healing service unlike any I had ever witnessed or experienced.

While Hurricane Harvey occurred almost seven years ago, the rebuilding is still ongoing. Many families have moved away, which has impacted their involvement and connection to our community. Home values and prices in the area have gone up as a result of the cost incurred in remediation, physically raising homes by six feet or more, and tak-ing other steps to prevent another catastrophe. These high costs and concerns about future disasters prevent many new families with young children from settling in our area.

Displacement is part of our Jewish heritage and legacy. We have been taught that we can find comfort and support through Torah and Jewish texts during times of suffering. As a community, we remained true to observing Shabbat and other sacred times throughout the rebuilding after Hurricane Harvey. We gathered together and found the important strength we needed to move forward.

Hurricanes are common in our area. However, through this storm, we learned how to be better prepared and to stay as safe as possible throughout the entire hurricane season. Improved drainage systems, wider bayou constructions, and other engineering steps have been taken to bring a sense of hope to this still traumatized community. With stronger foundations and elevated houses, we have found a way to live alongside the threat of natural disasters. We learn well from Psalms, which offers support and comfort during our most challenging moments. We are taught, "Hope in God, strengthen yourself, let your heart take courage, and hope in God" (Psalm 27:14).

We continue to thrive and grow as a faithful and spiritual community. Though Houston isn't perfect, it's a wonderful community that has been my home for the past twenty years. The unforgiving and tumultuous waters of Hurricane Harvey haven't deterred our spirit or our vision for a stronger, brighter, and drier future.

28

The Still, Small Voice
How Faith Helped Navigate California's Wildfires

RABBI PAUL KIPNES

A WILDFIRE burns out of control.

In the midst of the firestorm, burning its way through 96,949 acres, people asked, "Why is this happening?"

During the mandatory evacuation of more than 295,000 people, as they fled for their lives, people wondered, "Where is the protection we thought we were promised?"

Are these general questions or theological ones?

It seems that *during* the early phases of natural disasters like the wildfires that have been ravaging the American West and elsewhere, theological questions seem to surface only sporadically, even for those most faithful. We are too caught up in the confusion, too lost in the need to leave, and too worried to wonder about the whereabouts of our Maker.

But *after* the fires have substantially scorched the earth and *after* the fiery flames have incinerated our sense of personal safety, then, I find, people begin to cry out—at times in a heart-wrenching way, at times merely in a whisper—"And where was God?"

The Dichotomy Between "During" and "After"

That's the dichotomy between "during" and "after." During, we rush to survive. After, as we wander, we make time to wonder.

I believe that is what God wants us to do. When our Israelite ancestors stood on the shores of the Sea of Reeds—as Pharaoh's army threatened from behind and the sea blocked the way forward—our panicked people began praying. "Then God said to Moses, 'Why do you cry out to Me? Tell the Israelites to go forward" (Exodus 14:15).[1]

God advises us to set aside our theological thoughts during moments of danger. Instead, get moving! Later, after we and our loved ones are safe, or at least after the immediate danger has partially passed, then let's think about theology.

That was the wisdom that guided the experience of the Congregation Or Ami (Calabasas, California) community and our neighbors on November 8, 2018, when the Woolsey Fire ignited not far from the boundary between Los Angeles and Ventura Counties and quickly burned its way toward us.

A Community in Crisis

We were already a community in crisis. Eleven days before the Woolsey Fire, Congregation Or Ami—its congregants and clergy—like most Jewish communities, was reeling from the mass shooting at Pittsburgh's Tree of Life Synagogue. Ten days later, we faced a new tragedy: A gunman murdered many at the nearby Borderline Bar and Grill, a country-and-western dance bar frequented by our college and high school students. One of our Or Ami congregants narrowly escaped that carnage. Then, less than twenty-four hours after that, even before we had a chance to begin processing the shooting, the Woolsey Fire began.

The fear was intense. It was especially frightening for those of us with vivid memories of the October 2017 Tubbs Fire in Santa Rosa County (Northern California), which was, at the time, the most destructive wildfire in California history. That wildfire defied expectations, quickly and constantly changing directions, and endangered those who thought themselves safe from the fire's ferocity. Our Jewish community was still shocked and in mourning that the Tubbs Fire burned down our precious URJ Camp Newman in Santa Rosa, the summer camp that was home away from home for generations of Jewish youth.

The Woolsey Fire forced nearly 75 percent of our congregation to face mandatory evacuations. It destroyed 1,643 structures, including the homes of congregants and of our youth engagement coordinator.[2] The fires came so close to our synagogue's front door—about thirty feet away—that, fully expecting to lose our sacred home, my wife and I paused our volunteer work to say a distant goodbye to the building.

Sometime later the fires were contained and extinguished, and most of our evacuated congregants were back in their homes (*Hallelujah!*). Most—but not all. Thankfully, the fire spared the synagogue (*Praise God!*). Then as quickly as the fires arrived, the news cycle seemed to move on to the next tragedy.

The Trauma of "After"

Yet, for too many of our congregants and their neighbors, the trauma continued. Facing the fire's aftermath, we discovered that for those whose houses survived, the damage was still severe. A combination of smoke damage, toxic soot, and melted piping posed danger and required extensive remediation. The threat of mudslides also loomed from nearby denuded hillsides.

The extensive cleanup was complicated by continued crisis. People struggled to put their homes back together, calm their kids, and care for their folks. Fighting with insurance companies for repair authorizations that should have easily been approved sapped their strength. They were overwhelmed with the challenge of ascertaining finances, figuring out the permitting processes, and finding reputable repair teams.

Even those who made it through the fires ostensibly unscathed were struggling. One child showed up to our offsite religious school wearing oversized socks that turned out to be his father's because everything he owned still needed to be cleaned. Another child shed tears as she confessed she felt foolish in donated clothes. One mom was overwhelmed by the sheer volume of calls to banks, credit card companies, and insurance companies. Another dad was frustrated that the road ahead would be so long and arduous.

Now in the fire's aftermath, the initial appreciation for surviving gave way to a flood of complex feelings:

- The trauma of evacuation.
- The trauma of those mass shootings.
- The guilt that our homes survived while neighbors' homes had not.
- The worry that our sense of personal security was severely undermined.
- The anxiety that our children, parents, partners, and/or we ourselves would never really recover from that loss of security.

The wildfires had threatened us, and all indications showed that they would be back. Fires were now a regular part of Southern California life.

Seeking Solace After the Fires

Thus began "after": the second part of the story, when an evacuated community, having survived the fires and now wandering in the wilderness, began to embark on a soul-searing struggle to rediscover "Why?" Why did this happen to us, good people? Where was the protection promised us? Where was God?

Exhausted, still scared, reeling from the raw reality of what we went through, we needed something, anything that might help us cut through the cacophony to claim for ourselves calm, compassion, and a modicum of inner peace.

To many, it felt like God was absent. Even those unfamiliar with our nighttime *Hashkiveinu* prayer for protection knew that fundamental to our covenant with God is a basic agreement: The Holy One is supposed to spread a *sukkat shalom*, a "shelter of peace," over us. When that sukkah failed to appear, we wanted to know where and when we might find God again.

The Bible offers an explicit answer for times like this (I Kings 19:11–12):

> There was a great and mighty wind, splitting mountains and shattering rocks by God's power; but God was not in the wind. After the wind—an earthquake; but God was not in the earthquake. After the earthquake—fire; but God was not in the fire. And after the fire—a still, small voice.[3]

God, the Bible tells us, is not found in the hurricane winds, or the shaking earthquakes, or the uncontrollable wildfires. Don't look there—in the burning or the destruction, in the evacuations or your own trepidations. "Stop looking during those disasters," says the Holy One, "But afterward, when you're safe, do start listening. There you will find Me, in a still, small Voice, calling out to you. A Voice that was always present. Always whispering. Always inviting you to hear Me and feel My Presence."

These poignant words from our tradition remind us that during danger we should not get lost in theological thoughts. To follow our theological fancy while the fires are fast approaching would be a dangerous proposition. "Get moving!" God commands. "But then slow down and you will hear Me." That's what our tradition teaches: Survive now; ponder later.

So that's what we did in November 2018 when the Woolsey Fire endangered our community. We packed up and we fled; we supported and we fed the evacuees.

Sometimes, when it is hard to hear with our ears, we can just feel with our hearts. When the Torah was offered to our Israelite ancestors at Mount Sinai, our people responded, *Na'aseh v'nishma*, "We will do and [then] we will hear" (Exodus 24:7).[4] That became our mantra. *Now* we would act as we must, and hopefully the inner understanding—the "spiritual stuff" as one congregant called it—would follow *afterward*. So that's what we did. We heeded God's words, and only after did we seek God's Voice.

Slowing Down to Hear the Voice

As Jewish tradition promised, we eventually slowed down enough to hear the Voice. Surprisingly and with great satisfaction, we rediscovered that God had been right there with us—the evacuated and the exhausted—all along. God was in the kindness of strangers and in the compassionate actions of those never endangered, in the gift cards coming from across the country, and in the caring calls of colleagues and friends checking in for months to come.

It was not that God wasn't there during the fires; it was just that our "fight or flight" inner function forced us to choose. At first, during danger, we take flight. Later, after the immediate danger subsides, we fight our way back to renewed faith. And there we found the still, small Voice.

We heard the Holy One speaking to us in the wonderful words of those who hosted a Shabbat dinner for our community and felt the Holy Presence in the hugs of those who came by to hold us as we cried.

We voiced God's nearness through the four sets of phone calls we made to our community in the months afterward, and we imitated God's protective Presence through the professional-grade wildfire face masks we fundraised for and then handed out in the nearby firefighter staging camps.

We felt Holiness surrounding us. It was in whispered words of comfort to the kids who attended our pop-up Kids Camp and as we organized the community to care for those who lost their homes or felt like they were losing their minds.

During the *chanukat habayit* (rededication ceremony), which we celebrated on Shabbat Chanukah, we were finally able to bring our Torah scrolls back into our synagogue. We were buoyed by the standing-room-only crowd. As the voices sang out in full-throated faithfulness and praise, I recalled, with pleasure, the passage from our tradition:

> There was a great and mighty wind, splitting mountains and shattering rocks by God's power; but God was not in the wind. After the wind—an earthquake; but God was not in the earthquake. After the earthquake—fire; but God was not in the fire. And after the fire—a still, small voice.

Yes, after! Afterward, we heard that Voice. Just as God promised.

NOTES

1. Biblical translations are from *The JPS Tanakh: Gender-Sensitive Edition* (Jewish Publication Society, 2023), found on Sefaria (sefaria.org).
2. "After Action Review of the Woolsey Fire Incident," County of Los Angeles, https://file.lacounty.gov/SDSInter/bos/supdocs/144968.pdf.
3. The *JPS Tanakh* translates this phrase as "a soft murmuring sound," but it is often translated the way it appears here as "a still, small voice."
4. Translated by the author.

29

Choosing Life and Finding Resilience in the Face of AIDS

RABBI DENISE L. EGER

I WAS TWENTY-EIGHT years old. What did I really know about being a rabbi? What did I really know about death and dying? What did I really know about a disease without a cure? What did I really know about gay men and lesbians? What did I know about AIDS?

The answer: absolutely nothing.

But that is the world I entered as a newly ordained rabbi serving the world's first LGBTQ+ synagogue—Beth Chayim Chadashim—in 1988 during the height of the AIDS pandemic. It was a horrific time, when people with HIV/AIDS were diagnosed and then died within weeks. There were no medicines to treat HIV/AIDS and little understanding of the disease or how it was transmitted. There was so much fear. People feared getting it, feared those with it, and feared being "outed" as gay. After all, when AIDS was first noticed, it was called the "gay cancer" or "GRID" (gay-related immune deficiency). Because the outbreak of AIDS first spread rapidly in the gay male community—a community already stigmatized and ostracized by society—the stigma of having AIDS was immeasurable. Christian fundamentalists routinely voiced that AIDS was a punishment from God for being gay. Under President Ronald Reagan's administration, and subsequently under President George H. W. Bush's administration, countless people with AIDS died because the government did nothing; in fact, they did worse than nothing—they often prevented the Centers for Disease Control from helping. A *New York Times* article by Jeffrey Schmalz in August 1992 states, "The epidemic was more than five years old before President Ronald Reagan uttered the 'A' word publicly."[1]

It was a time when families rejected their children for being gay or lesbian, and longtime lovers and partners had no legal protections. Gay and lesbian people stayed in the closet for fear of losing their jobs and housing. So great was this fear that even in our LGBTQ+ synagogue, most members didn't use their last names. And all of the trauma still lives in me, as it does in many in the LGBTQ+ community who lived through those early years of the AIDS pandemic: the fear and trauma of further rejection, of infection, or of being outed; the trauma of losing all of our friends and chosen family in great numbers. We lived with layers upon layers of grief and loss, illness, and overwhelming helplessness.

During that time, week in and week out, I would travel from hospital to hospital across the vast freeways of Los Angeles County. I would visit AIDS patients as they lay dying, sometimes very alone, with no family in sight. In those early years, several of the hospitals had AIDS floors or AIDS wards. I would just go from bed to bed to offer a hand and a cheerful smile, sometimes to feed patients who no longer had the strength to feed themselves, and always to offer a blessing. Having grown up in a more classical Reform tradition, I had never heard of the *Mi Shebeirach* prayer for healing until rabbinical school. I quickly learned that I needed something authentic from my own tradition to say at those moments. Sometimes I offered a *Mi Shebeirach* for healing at the bedside if there was hope, and sometimes it was the *Vidui*, the Final Confession, if they were in the final stages of death.

I had recited the *Vidui*, the confessional prayer, only at the end of Yom Kippur services, but now I was reciting it at the bedside of dying Jewish AIDS patients. If they were able to speak, I helped them recite it. What did it mean to be forgiven of their sins in a world that called gay men sinful? Yet here were beautiful young men, who lived their lives with dignity and integrity, dying from a disease that had no cure or vaccine. The sin was not theirs but ours, in how the world was mistreating LGBTQ+ people and specifically people with AIDS. But more often than not, by the time I arrived, I was reciting it for them.

The healing prayer took on a powerful, almost magical meaning. We restored the *Mi Shebeirach* to our Reform Jewish liturgy because of the AIDS pandemic. During Shabbat services, it became part of the regular liturgical practice. Service leaders would read a list of names of those who were ill or ask for names to be said aloud. Just as the congregation would rise to say the Mourner's *Kaddish* in memory of those lesbian and gay people who had no one to say *Kaddish* for them, we added for "those who died of AIDS." This was the start of how we dealt with the trauma of those years. We spoke the truth about AIDS. People died.

Talking with other colleagues serving LGBTQ+ Jewish communities in other cities, we collaboratively worked on compiling healing services and prayers to be recited bedside. Rabbi Janet Marder, who preceded me at Beth Chayim Chadashim, began the work. Then Rabbi Yoel Kahn in San Francisco and I were simultaneously offering weekly healing services separate from Shabbat worship. They became community support and grief groups that helped people with AIDS (when they weren't too weak to attend) have some hope. Those who witnessed the decimation happening in their midst attended as well. Friends and family, both chosen and biological, attended; some doctors and nurses who were treating those with HIV/AIDS attended; coworkers and neighbors of those who were ill and dying of AIDS attended. Synagogue members were quickly realizing that AIDS wasn't something happening "out there" to others but existed within our own temple and community. Overcoming the denial of AIDS as a Jewish issue was a critical first step. We were bringing AIDS out of the synagogue closet and into the open.

These weekly healing services gave birth to a specific support group for people with HIV/AIDS. There was as much shame within the synagogue about members' HIV statuses as there was in the outside world, and many people did not want their name on the healing list. They suffered from the prevalent shame of being HIV positive. And yet, people who were newly diagnosed had unique issues they needed to share, and they craved the support and learning that could only be found with one another.

Perhaps it was my naivete and youth that led me to believe I could facilitate such a group. It certainly wasn't the only HIV support group in town. However, two temple members with HIV came to me and said their needs as Jews weren't being met in other groups. So we gathered every other week, and the group members would share their concerns, stories, information about the latest medical and political news, or remembrances of those lovers and friends who had died. They grieved for themselves and their situations, and they grieved for their many friends who were dead or dying. It was and still is unimaginable and overwhelming.

So we agreed that during each meeting, everyone would also share something positive. Maybe it was only that they were able to get out of bed that day. Maybe it was that someone had the courage to share their status with a family member. Maybe it was that they had a nice date. This emphasis on positivity helped focus our conversations and transform them into an antidote to the trauma. Viktor Frankl's tragic optimism, as described in his book *Man's Search for Meaning* as the ability to experience optimism even in times of untold suffering, was a guide for our support group and for me.

In our support groups, I also taught Torah. Each session I tried to find something in our tradition to bring hope and comfort. Sometimes I taught from the *parashah* (Torah portion) and sometimes from a text related to an upcoming holiday. Sometimes we interpreted and reinterpreted the meaning of a ritual or idea. Teaching Torah as a rabbi was something I knew how to do, and it helped me address the trauma of leading at such a time. But teaching Torah to a group of gay men who often had little or no Jewish education was a challenge; teaching Torah to a group of gay men who also had been raised to be ashamed of their sexuality, who had often been kicked out of their Jewish communities or families because they were gay, and who were taught to be further ashamed because they now had AIDS was yet another challenge.

We met these challenges by focusing on Jewish ideals. *Uvacharta bachayim*, "Therefore choose life" (Deuteronomy 30:19), became part of our mantra—choosing to live rather than simply give in to what was then a death sentence. Building friendships and camaraderie in the group helped to stem the tide of social isolation that accompanied a diagnosis. I encouraged them to attend Shabbat services, and they did, sitting together, even when they had deep doubts about God or great anger at the God they didn't believe in. We created a new understanding of the Chanukah story: they became the jar of oil that lasted longer than anyone expected. We studied midrashim about the broken set of the Ten Commandments that still were sacred and held in the Holy Ark, and I made explicit the understanding that though they felt broken, they were holy—holy enough to be held in the most sacred divine spaces. They wrapped themselves in tallitot, imagining it as an embrace of God, even when the preachers on TV told them they were sinners.

For me, finding and mining our tradition for new insights that could affirm their humanity and dignity and give them hope helped me cope as well. This support group continued even as I began a new congregation in the Los Angeles area, and I continued to lead it for another thirty years, offering a safe Jewish space for those with HIV/AIDS, welcoming the newly diagnosed, and even occasionally welcoming non-Jews who needed spiritual grounding to cope with being HIV positive. Sometimes straight folks with HIV joined. Of course, we mourned each member of the group who died during those many years.

World AIDS Day observances became a holy day for both remembrance and education. To help mark this day Jewishly, I created readings and prayers to be shared for the occasion, which is commemorated annually on December 1. Adapting the Jewish tradition of lighting a *yahrzeit* candle, we lit red votive candles, because wearing a red ribbon became a symbol of honoring those with HIV/AIDS and remembering those who died.[2] We displayed the NAMES Project AIDS Memorial Quilt[3] panels, which was a response to the overwhelming trauma and loss due to HIV/AIDS. I also organized annual interfaith gatherings for World AIDS Day that included elected officials, long-term survivors, and the doctors and educators who were some of the earliest caretakers of people with HIV and who carried their own trauma of those years. Arranging these observances was also a way to help me cope with my own trauma. We created a safe space and fostered collaboration among health-care professionals, community leaders, those living with HIV, and those grieving someone who died from HIV/AIDS. By having members of the HIV/AIDS support group help plan and speak at this annual gathering, I encouraged them to focus on their strengths and resilience as long-term survivors. When they shared their stories and struggles, it helped shape the synagogue into a trauma-informed organization. Prayer, *tzedakah*, Torah, memorializing, community building, coalition building, advocacy, and education all were and remain aspects of coping with the losses.

The most enduring of my memories that remain part of the trauma that lives in me are of standing at grave after grave and burying young men my own age or barely older than me. Whenever I visit those cemeteries, I try to visit many of those graves; some haven't had a single other visitor since the funeral. I know I am the bearer of memory for many of these young people who died way too early in their lives from a disease that few cared about and many still do not care about. I think of them at *Yizkor* each year, and I keep a list of their names, lest I forget.

In 1978, only a few years before five gay men in Los Angeles would be reported to be sick with pneumocystis pneumonia (an infection that would become highly associated with HIV/AIDS), Harvey Milk addressed the rally at the San Francisco Gay Freedom Day Parade from the steps of San Francisco City Hall. Milk, who in 1977 became the first openly gay person elected to public office in California, spoke about the most important thing for those who experienced discrimination, particularly LGBTQ+ people. His assassination in November of 1978 spurred a revolution of activism in the LGBTQ+ community. As AIDS began to wreak havoc in San Francisco and in gay communities just a few years after his death, that activism would transform and inspire the LGBTQ+ community in taking care of our own people when the world shunned those ill with AIDS because of government inaction and malfeasance. Milk's emphasis on hope in spite of the difficulties and attacks on LGBTQ+ people remains an inspiration today just as it inspired the early AIDS activists: "The only thing they have to look forward to is hope. And you have to give them hope. Hope for a better world, hope for a better tomorrow, hope for a better place to come to if the pressures at home are too great. Hope that all will be all right. Without hope, not only gays, but the blacks, the seniors, the handicapped, the us'es, the us'es will give up."[4]

We didn't give up, despite the pain, sadness, suffering, and overwhelming illnesses. The people with AIDS, the long-term survivors, didn't give up. Instead, through Jewish tradition and innovation, community building, and the age-old emphasis on hope in Jewish tradition—even in the darkest hours—we ultimately found our mechanism for dealing with trauma.

NOTES

1. Jeffrey Schmalz, "Republicans Face an AIDS Test," *New York Times*, August 16, 1992.

2. In 1991, nearly a decade after the discovery of AIDS, a group of New York artists got together to work on a visual AIDS project. They were inspired by the yellow ribbons used to support the military fighting in the Gulf War. These artists partnered with Broadway Cares and Equity Fights AIDS to have guests and presenters wear red ribbons at the June 1991 Tony Awards. The Broadway community had been deeply affected by AIDS losses.

3. Conceived by LGBTQ+ activist Cleve Jones in 1985, the AIDS Memorial Quilt was made up of panels created by individuals across the United States and Canada to memorialize friends and family members who died of HIV/AIDS. It was displayed numerous times in Washington, DC, on the National Mall but has grown too large to show in its entirety. For more information or to display a section of the quilt, visit www.aidsmemorial.org.

4. Harvey Milk's Gay Freedom Day Parade Speech, June 25, 1978, https://www.docsteach.org/documents/document/milk-hope-speech.

30

Nachamu Ami, Comfort My People

Serving as a Hospital Chaplain During COVID

Rabbi Leah Cohen Tenenbaum, DMin, BCC, PCAHC

It was March of 2020. We were gathered around the table in the conference room. Our interdisciplinary team of doctors, advanced practice providers, residents, fellows, nurses, social workers, and the chaplain meets daily to discuss each patient on the palliative care list. Palliative care is a consult service at the hospital that provides an additional layer of support for seriously ill patients. That day, our morning routine began as usual, familiar faces, sipping our normal morning beverages, and a bit of kibitzing. Then we began to run the list, going over each name, relevant medical information, and plan for the day for that patient, when suddenly someone pointed out a new column on the spreadsheet generated from the electronic medical records.

We were all silent and wore quizzical expressions. People pulled out their Mobile Heartbeat hospital cell phones, but no announcements had been made.

We would all get to know this new column intimately in the next few months, as its numbers and impact overwhelmed not just our spreadsheet, but every aspect of the hospital's ecosystem. This new column was one you never wanted to see marked with an X next to a name. It meant that the patient had tested positive for COVID-19. But in that meeting, all we could do was naively ask, "What's this?"

The question "What have we learned?" has been evolving ever since we awoke to COVID-19. Though much changed during the pandemic, our lasting lessons remain elusive. Although we have made some impressive scientific breakthroughs, especially around infectious diseases, I have been underwhelmed by any advances in the moral or social realms. In fact, the greatest learning for me has been that ancient Jewish teachings are the most enduring source of guidance, resilience, and wisdom in this brave new world.

My role on the palliative care team at a large academic hospital is to address issues of spiritual and existential distress for patients, families, and staff. This process has three parts:

1. Assess the situation.
2. Implement the appropriate interventions.
3. Integrate those spiritual interventions into the plan of care by collaborating with the primary, specialty, and palliative care teams.

Assessment

Kol haolam kulo gesher tzar m'od, v'ha-ikar lo l'facheid k'lal, "The whole world is a very narrow bridge, but the main thing is to have no fear at all" (Rabbi Nachman of Bratzlav, *Likutei Moharan* 2:48:2:7).

In the hospital setting, illness, pain, suffering, and death coexist with the pursuit of health, compassion, comfort, and hope. Fear lurks in the background, but it is something we assess for and address using our professional resources. Is a patient afraid of experiencing pain? Let us have our experts in pain management come in. Is a family afraid of financial insecurity? We will have our social worker speak with you. Afraid of going to hell after you die? Our chaplain will be by. If we detect a patient fears returning home, we will assess for a safe discharge and generate a plan. Fear is just one of many things we assess for and address in a variety of ways.

But this was different. During the height of COVID, fear was not only coming from patients and their families; it was also coming from frontline staff and management. We feared not knowing how to allocate resources, keep staff safe, address shortages, or calculate the next steps. We were afraid of getting sick or infecting our families, yet most of us felt called to this work for deeply moral reasons, and some financially needed to work. The world had become a very narrow bridge, and frankly, people were starting to fall off.

One of the most difficult aspects of this new reality was the way fear creates isolation. The virus, by necessity, required isolation. However, the hospital quickly recognized that COVID would be a battle for both patients and the staff offering care. No one could fight this battle alone, so early on, the hospital borrowed the military concept of the "buddy system" to help the staff survive under all the stress and isolation.

Everyone who worked at the hospital coped with COVID in their own way. Some left their jobs, found permanent ways to work from home, or came in but hid. Some had to care for family members or got sick themselves. But for those who stepped up to the front line, the buddy system was key. With a buddy, you can cross a narrow bridge, hand in hand.

I had a buddy. She was brave and funny. We sent each other snarky text messages and ate our lunch on a bench outside when we could. We listened to each other, comforted each other, and always had each other's backs. Then one day, she had had enough. I saw the pressure building, but I could always find a way to make her laugh, even as the insanity, injustice, and tension rose. For so many on the front line, the adrenaline of dealing with what was in front of us got us through the next thing we had to do.

For some of the staff, it was what happened after the peak of COVID that was their final straw. My buddy left, as did others, during the efforts to transition back to "normal" at the hospital. As rules and regulations switched multiple times, trust and communication often gave way to confusion and frustration, which compounded the trauma of the COVID experience. My buddy and I are still in touch, however, and each text message still begins, "Hi Buddy."

Dazed a bit, I stayed, putting one foot in front of the other, wading through the uncertainties, pivoting, dodging, and taking the hands of those who remained to continue across the narrow bridge. Gradually, I navigated the "new normal" and my fear gave way to acceptance.

Interventions

Ometz lev (courage).

I have always appreciated the etymology of the Hebrew phrase for "courage." Sure, we can hear the Latin *coer* and know that courage has something to do with the heart in English. But the Hebrew for "courage," *ometz lev*, literally means "exertions of the heart." People ask me, "What exactly does a hospital chaplain do?" Especially during the pandemic, the most accurate answer would be: exertions of the heart. Chaplains are trained in spiritual interventions. We function as a non-anxious presence by actively listening, advocating for patients, and offering prayers, rituals, and religious material. We facilitate conversations around goals of care, supporting patients and families from diagnosis to end of life, educating staff on spiritual matters, and addressing moral distress. Regardless of one's training, experience, and resources, what these spiritual interventions all require is action and compassion. If that's not exertion of the heart, I don't know what is.

One story that illustrates this exertion of the heart took place shortly after the peak of COVID when visitor restrictions had been lifted. One day I was up in the cardiothoracic intensive care unit (CTICU). A patient was about to be removed from the life-support equipment that had been keeping her heart going. In addition to her cardiac issues, she had some family dynamics that I imagine had also taken a toll. The patient's significant other had been alternatively on and off visitor restrictions due to the family's wishes and his agitated behavior on the floor. However, it had been decided that he would be allowed to visit for this final act, as she was expected to pass imminently.

The family gathered around her bedside, and I was called in to provide end-of-life support. As I took in the tearful family encircling the patient, I saw out of the corner of my eye that security had also been notified. The armed guards discreetly gathered outside the room.

The physician came in. Young, bespeckled, and anxious, he began to explain the next steps. The gentleman of concern stood apart. As the family quietly nodded their understanding, he raised his voice, "What are you doing? I will not allow this. God will save her. You cannot do this." The doctor attempted to explain in a calm voice how we had reached this moment. The family froze. Tension was rising. I knew I had to act quickly.

I strode across the room and gently put my arm around his shoulders. I boldly declared, "I stand with you in faith!" Silence. The machines sighed; the humans exhaled. "Come on," I said to my new buddy, "let's get outta here." I escorted him to get some water, then down to the lobby and out the door, all while speaking words of comfort. Eventually, he settled down and left the hospital peacefully. When I returned to the floor, one of the security guards said, "How did you do that?" I put my arm around his shoulder and looked him in the eyes, "Gentle touch and faith affirmation. And God loves you too."

Plan of Care

Nachamu, nachamu ami (Isaiah 40:1).

This famous supplication can be translated as "Comfort my people, comfort them." But who is giving this comfort, who are "my people," and what exactly is "comfort"? Most days, Isaiah's words feel like a job description to me. "My people" are all the names on the palliative care consult list, regardless of religion, race, age, gender, socioeconomic or legal status.

"Comfort," in this setting, has so many nuances. Pain management is a form of comfort. But with a terminal illness, the word "comfort" takes on new meanings. In the beginning, treatment and pain management are usually pursued simultaneously. However, as the disease progresses, diagnostics are set aside, treatment options are exhausted, and the objective becomes to make the patient as comfortable as possible as they approach the end of life.

During the height of COVID, our hospital ran into a difficult comfort problem. Usually, once a person's plan of care has transitioned to focus on comfort measures only (CMO), they are transferred to hospice. However, hospice was initially not able to handle the waves of COVID patients. Patients were admitted to the hospital for serious complications from COVID; many were not getting better, so they would transition to CMO, then hospice. At that time, there was no place for them to physically go. They could not stay on the main hospital floors, because we needed the beds for patients who required active treatment. We were dangerously low on staff and supplies. Hospice patients couldn't go home, and visitor restrictions were in place. They had to leave, but there was no place to send them.

Thus, the supportive care unit was born. We took over an area of the hospital and set up our own end-of-life unit for COVID positive patients who were CMO. Our sole purpose was to provide comfort for those who were going to die from COVID in the hospital.

One of the most impactful elements that I incorporated in this setting was something I called "door bios." I interviewed families, talked to the patient (if possible), and gathered input from the staff. Then I wrote a one-page summary in a narrative, first-person voice based on the material I collected. I hung the door bio on the patient's sealed door so anyone entering would have a more humanized vision of the person and situation they were about to encounter. I read the bios to the families. They asked for copies. These pieces became part of the families' legacies—as well as mine. This was one way I could build bridges of trust to improve our therapeutic relationship in a time of so much fear, despair, and distrust.

I journeyed back and forth across these bridges. I met a daughter at the hospital entrance who delivered a small Buddha statue to place near her mother's bed. I printed pictures families emailed me and hung them in their loved one's rooms. I listened to a son express his guilt over not getting vaccinated, infecting his father, and now watching his father die. They brought me their grief, their objects, their love. I brought them empathy, dignity, and acceptance. Even when family could not be with their loved ones due to visitor restrictions, no one died alone. With the use of iPads and WhatsApp, with pictures and stories, with the gentle hands and presence of staff, no one was abandoned in their final hour.

Trauma Informed Care Through a Jewish Lens

Today the pandemic is yesterday's news, though every year new strains emerge, patients are admitted to the hospital, and some still die. There are so many aftereffects—not just the physical effects of "long COVID," but the possibly more impactful trauma this pandemic bequeathed us. Trauma can rob us of our sense of agency, wholeness, and autonomy.

I think about trauma informed care through the lens of our morning prayer: *Modeh/modah ani l'fanecha, Melech chai v'kayam, shehechezarta bi nishmati b'chemlah. Rabah emunatecha*, "I offer thanks to You, ever-living Sovereign, that You have restored my soul to me in mercy: How great is Your trust in me." What an empowering statement! Even with all the brokenness of this pandemic, God trusts us. The Almighty thinks we've got this! I draw strength from this audacious idea.

How do we deliver on God's faith in us? In small ways. We've all heard the phrase "The devil is in the details." This is true when I think about the administrative aspects of my job or the challenges of collaborating on complex cases. But Judaism offers another perspective that rings truer for me: *Elohim b'pratim*, "The Divine is in the details." When I pause to listen to a tearful resident share her first patient death or coordinate moving a patient's bed closer to the window so he can wave to his seven-year-old daughter on her birthday, I feel sure that God has orchestrated these details.

At my core, I have an underlying philosophy grounded in my Judaism that keeps me going: "One who visits a sick person takes away one-sixtieth of their illness" (Babylonian Talmud, *Bava M'tzia* 30b). The idea is that one's visit lightens the sick person's suffering. Why by one-sixtieth? That seems like such a tiny amount! But one-sixtieth is a symbolic number that represents a tipping point. It comes from the rules of kashrut. If milk and meat come into contact with each other, the food is rendered unkosher and cannot be eaten. How much mixing would it take to make something kosher become unkosher? The Rabbis ruled that even a drop of milk would make a pot of meat stew inedible (Babylonian Talmud, *Chulin* 108a). How much is a drop? One sixtieth of the volume of the stew (*Mishneh Torah*, Forbidden Foods, 9:9). One-sixtieth is a tiny bit, but it changes everything.

The problems of this pandemic and the health-care system are so much larger than I am. But if I can hold up an iPad and decrease someone's loneliness by one-sixtieth, or recite a blessing and increase a person's hope by one-sixtieth, if I can help families overcome their grief by one-sixtieth or teach a resident how to communicate with his patients better by one-sixtieth, or help a nurse finish her shift with the last one-sixtieth of her compassion, then what was inedible becomes edible and what was unbearable becomes bearable. Then I have fulfilled my obligation, I have been of use, and together we have crossed the narrow bridge.

PART FIVE

Trauma and Community

31

The Legacy of Trauma

Reckoning with the Reform Movement's Ethical Misconduct

RABBI MARINA YERGIN

I AM A PRODUCT of the Reform Movement. I grew up in a Reform congregation, attended a Reform camp, participated in Reform youth groups. When I knew at age twelve that I wanted to become a rabbi, the only option I entertained was to attend the Reform Movement's seminary, Hebrew Union College–Jewish Institute of Religion (HUC-JIR). For most of my life, the Reform Movement brought me pride.

It also brought me sadness. Fear. Anger. Hurt. You see, I am one of the survivors of the Reform Movement's ethical misconduct. This is my story.

In 2000, when I was a camper at a Union for Reform Judaism (URJ) camp, I was sexually abused by a counselor. I didn't know anything was wrong until a fellow camper raised concern. It was then that I learned that I was not the only female camper this male counselor was grooming. Once I and others reported it to a different counselor, things snowballed and he was fired.

Soon after, I remember sitting in the dark with everyone in a circle crying. The boys were mad at the girls because their favorite counselor was gone. I remember the camp's director and associate director sitting on chairs in front of the fireplace to talk to us. I remember there being conversations about how what had happened was sexual assault or sexual harassment. I distinctly remember being told by the director that none of that was true: There was no assault. There was no harassment. I believed him. I was eleven.

For years, I slept with my door open and made my parents open theirs as well, because there were rumors going around that the counselor in question had a copy of the camp's roster that had all of our contact information, and he was going to come and hurt all of us because we got him fired. I had nightmares that would wake me up screaming because of what he did to me and other campers. For years, I would ask trusted adults about the definitions of and difference between sexual harassment and sexual abuse to try to clarify what had happened to me and why people whom I thought were trusted adults had lied.

The next summer I returned to camp and had to be dragged out of the car. The fear and pain didn't go away, but I pushed it aside because I wanted to fit in. I wanted to be at the place that I considered home. I wanted to be with my friends. I wanted to grow Jewishly. I do strongly believe that my thirteen years at this URJ camp helped define me as a person and as a rabbi. At the same time, this dark spot on my time at this URJ camp remains in my memory and in my heart. I did not believe that any of this would resurface the way it did, but in 2021 the Reform Movement would be faced with its movement-wide and generation-spanning history of ethical misconduct. I definitely didn't think that as a result of the process, I would endure additional trauma.

It began in April 2021, when two rabbis' ethical misconduct was widely reported by survivors. These reports then led to investigations by multiple Reform institutions: the URJ, the Central Conference of American Rabbis (CCAR), HUC-JIR, and three Reform synagogues. All three Reform Movement institutions (URJ, CCAR, and HUC-JIR) hired independent law firms to investigate misconduct.

When it was announced that there were going to be independent law firms investigating harms, I knew I had to speak out about my own experience. During my interview with the law firm hired by the URJ, I reported my story. I knew that the counselor had been fired, but—as I found out through this investigation—he was never reported to the police nor was his conduct reported to the URJ. I was devastated to learn that I experienced not only the original harm done by this man, but also secondary harm by the director and associate director for not reporting the harm-doer and his actions to the URJ or the police. To prepare for my interview with the law firm, I chose to contact some of the counselors and the unit head from that summer to make sure that my eleven-year-old self's memory was accurate. My memories were corroborated, and I could see the deep trauma that others also carried from being bystanders and not having sufficient tools or guidance at that time to help me or the other campers. During the time I was interviewed by the URJ investigators, each institution was conducting their own interviews and compiling reports.

All three institutional reports were later released publicly.[1] The investigations and subsequent reports aimed to be transparent about harms done in the institutions and give suggestions for some resolutions. The reports, particularly the ones regarding the URJ and HUC-JIR,[2] highlighted years of misconduct in many categories. There was an overarching theme of a violation of boundaries—sexual, educational, intellectual, emotional, professional, and so on. These egregious harms included but were not limited to sexual abuse and sexual harassment; blackmail; gaslighting; child sexual abuse; psychological harm; emotional harm; physical harm; hiding harms known to institutions and institutional leadership; lack of reporting harms to institutions, parents, and/or law enforcement; and abuse of a role of power to perpetrate more harms. The reported misconduct impacted people of all identities but was more intense for those in marginalized groups—Jews of Color, members of the LGBTQIA+ community, and women. Each report finished with a section of recommendations for further work to stop future harm, support survivors, and implement new policies to guide the institutions and help survivors. Each institution decided which of these recommendations they would pursue. These reports only scratch the surface of the deep trauma found in the Reform Movement for generations.

The HUC-JIR report, compiled by the law firm Morgan Lewis, was thirty-seven pages and was released in November 2021.[3] It covered a wide range of findings and observations including naming six harm-doers—most of whom were deceased or already known due to press reports. The CCAR report, compiled by the law firm Alcalaw, was eighty-four pages and was released in December 2021; it focused solely on the CCAR ethics process.[4] The URJ report, assembled by the law firm Debevoise & Plimpton, was 121 pages long and was released in February 2022.[5] The report named some harm-doers and focused on the many different facets that make up the URJ— conferences, camps, youth programs, human resources, and so on. The appendixes section focused on the existing policies and codes of conduct.

In many cases, the reports laid out both specific details and general overviews of the trauma experienced by the survivors. However, it is imperative to highlight that in asking the survivors to come forward and share their stories, they were being asked to relive their trauma with strangers without knowing the outcome. It may have been the first time or the millionth time someone shared the harm they endured, but restating it and reliving it bring its own kind of trauma.

For example, I also made a report as part of the HUC-JIR process, and the interview left me feeling like I was a harm-doer because I didn't directly report or recognize the harms in the moment they were happening. The amount of guilt that came from the interview where I was putting my career and safety on the line was extremely detrimental to me.

Fortunately, there are things that the reports and institutions got right. Some survivors felt that the reports demonstrated that that their trauma was finally being recognized and that they could share it with their family and friends. Each institution also took actionable steps to repair harm. HUC-JIR offered to reissue diplomas so that the names of harm-doers would not be permanently etched there. They also offered a new ordination for those who wanted it and hired a director of *t'shuvah* (repentance) to help guide some of these opportunities.

In response to recommendations in the CCAR report, the Ethics Process Review Committee revised the ethics code. The CCAR created the Task Force on Ethics to find ways to improve the process and hired an ethics advisor for inquiries and complaint intake. The CCAR invited the wider community to take part in confidential *t'shuvah* conversations with the organization's leadership, and many chose to do so, including individuals, family members, and congregational leadership. In addition, CCAR leadership reached out to individuals who had been harmed and institutions where harm had occurred in the 1970s and 1980s, before there was an ethics code, for private *t'shuvah*-focused conversations and institutional apologies. The CCAR was also the first of the Reform institutions to create a *t'shuvah* ritual for the High Holy Days 5782/2021 using Yom Kippur liturgy. It was led by rabbis of diverse backgrounds and recognized the wrongs that have been done over the years CCAR has existed.

The URJ created task forces and working groups to think through various aspects of the process such as congregational ethics codes, restorative justice, and more. The URJ later hired Dr. Guila Benchimol and Dr. Alissa Ackerman of Ampersands Restorative Justice to work on a restorative justice process. Rabbi Rick Jacobs, the president of the URJ, created a Yom Kippur amends video, and a *Mi Shebeirach* (prayer of healing) for survivors was delivered at the URJ's 150th anniversary event in December 2023.[6]

That being said, there are areas where I believe the reports missed the mark. While some of the institutions were clear that everyone was invited to share their stories, there was some ambiguity, and some people—such as family members of those harmed, upstanders, bystanders, family members of the wrongdoers, and witnesses—did not feel welcome to participate. The reports also caused secondary trauma— trauma not resulting from initial harm. For example, the reports made some realize that they were bystanders in the harmful situations they witnessed. Others have expressed concern that some individuals with important information may have self-excluded and did not participate, feeling misconduct was not their story to tell if they weren't a direct survivor. Many survivors chose not to participate for fear of reexperiencing their own trauma or of retribution, even though the law firms made it clear that retribution was prohibited.

In addition, the impact on survivors' Judaism can be profound. Some individuals have sought a different stream of Judaism or even left the Jewish world. Some cited their trauma as the primary reason for their changed connection to Judaism. Indeed, places they thought would be safe ruined their entire understanding of Judaism and of safety. These realizations have also caused generations of harm, as parents have chosen to remove their children from Jewish spaces because they do not believe them to be safe. Sadly, this means that a number of people who could have spoken to the investigators were not aware of the investigations. Unless they were currently involved in the Reform Movement, many individuals may not even have known the investigations were happening and therefore lost the opportunity to share their experience.

That said, the investigators did hear from some individuals who were no longer involved in the Reform Movement.

For months after the reports were released, the institutions' communication about next steps varied. In some cases, committees were formed and new policies were drafted. I and other survivors perceived a lack of communication and action. A grassroots effort—led by a group called ACT (Accountable, Community-focused, Transparent)—disseminated a letter "demand[ing] swift and meaningful action in response to the . . . URJ Ethics Investigation Report."[7] In a matter of days, the letter had over five hundred signatories. A few weeks later, I was contacted by one of the organizers of ACT asking me, as clergy, to write an email to Rabbi Rick Jacobs and then Board Chair Jennifer Brodkey Kaufman. I shared with them my own experience—the same experience I shared at the beginning of this chapter.

I received feedback almost immediately from the URJ leadership, which led to individual Zoom meetings and an invitation to be on a working group for restorative justice. Over a year later, my persistence and communication resulted in me, a survivor, serving on the URJ ethics leadership team to be able to give that perspective—my perspective. It was intimidating to feel like I had to represent every survivor as the survivor in those meetings, and it took me a long time to really step forward with my survivor role as front and center. By doing so, I was able to finally speak for my eleven-year-old self.

One of the most important elements of this process is the concept of institutional harm. Institutional harm is the mistreatment of a person by a system of power, and it is different from the primary harm that occurred. When institutions cause additional harm based on their silence and lack of accountability, ethical misconduct is perpetuated and harms continue. It may be that current leadership of these institutions is not connected to the original harm-doers or the primary harm; still, in order to be fully accountable and prevent ongoing trauma, institutions must take seriously their roles as perpetuators of harm. As many people struggle with the trauma caused by these institutional harms, it is common for survivors to be silenced. However, we learn that it is a Jewish value to express rebuke in a kind, thoughtful, and direct way. It is not done as a punishment, but so that our institutions understand what has happened and can improve. As Rabbi Danya Ruttenberg says in her book *On Repentance and Repair: Making Amends in an Unapologetic World*, "rebuke is a call to accountability."[8]

How, then, do we understand this accountability? The answer can be found in *Hilchot T'shuvah*, the Laws of Repentance laid out by Maimonides in his *Mishneh Torah*, a legal compendium written in the late twelfth century.[9] These laws explain how to go through a *t'shuvah* process with another person by following five steps. The steps are unique to Judaism in the way they are laid out, and it is noted that the entire five-step process must be survivor-focused and survivor-engaged or it is not being done correctly.

First, the harm-doer must name and own the harm. Even before this step, the harm-doer must understand the harm they have caused and be willing to face it, many times in a public arena. This public statement of ownership is not an apology; it is a recognition of the harm, with full ownership and a commitment to engage in the process of transformation.

The second step is to change their behavior, showing commitment to the process of *t'shuvah* and transformation. It may seem odd that there is no apology made at this step, but Maimonides explains that this step is about transformation, an outer reflection of the inner effort that must be done before the harm-doer can move forward in the repentance process. The harm-doer should focus on bettering themselves—delving into the root causes of the harm, going to therapy or rehab, or educating themselves.

The third step is restitution and accepting consequences.[10] Before jumping into this step, we must be willing to talk to survivors and understand what restitution they need. Dr. Guila Benchimol, who worked on the URJ's restorative justice process, explains that amends are not gifts to be offered to or with those harmed,[11] but are what the harm-doer owes those harmed.[12] The survivor has the right to decide what kind of restitution they are seeking—restitution must be survivor-centered.

The fourth step is apology. For many people, this will seem late in the game. However, Maimonides reminds us that it must be one of the last steps to prove it is authentic and the result of true transformation and understanding. Again, the focus is on the survivor. What kind of apology do they need? What actions has the harm-doer undertaken to be able to apologize in a wholehearted, transformed way? Rabbi Ruttenberg highlights that "a real apology is not aimed at the person who has been hurt, but rather is given in relationship with them."[13]

The fifth and final step is that when and if the harm-doer is faced with the same situation, they make a different choice. This is evidence of their efforts to understand the harm they caused and the ways they have changed. This also means that at any point—a week, a year, fifty years—a person could be faced with the same situation and must make a different choice. In other words, the work of *t'shuvah* never really ends.

Some of this is being done in our institutions, and each organization is at a different step. As time passes, each of the institutions and survivors are learning more about *t'shuvah* and the restorative justice process. They are learning what it means to be truly survivor-centered. They may still miss the mark in various ways, but we are learning together and moving forward.

As Rabbi Ruttenberg says, the reality is "we cannot change the past, yet we can change the future, but only if we are honest about what has been—and who was harmed, and who caused that harm."[14] We can no longer think someone else will take up the hard work. We cannot ignore misconduct of any kind and think that there will not be anyone impacted by it. We must realize that when we don't stand up against misconduct, we are secondary harm-doers, causing even more harm to the survivor.

It is not a matter of if, but when the next instance of ethical misconduct will occur. This is the reality of our world and human nature. The only thing that will help is that we need to have structures in place throughout the entire Reform Movement that will be our new norm. These must be integrated into who we are as Reform Jews, as a community. We can only do that if we own our past and the problems it has caused for generations.

NOTES

1. The Women's Rabbinic Network (WRN) has collated all the reports and other documentation at www.wrnresources.org. The WRN created this website to centralize the accountability and repair information of the

Reform Movement to support victim-survivors and ensure good, quality communication. The WRN, with the leadership of Rabbi Mary Zamore, WRN's executive director, has been instrumental in this work and has been advocating for survivors for a long time—before the ethics investigations even began.

2. CCAR's investigation and therefore the resulting report focused on their ethics process. The URJ and HUC-JIR's investigations invited reports of all and any type of harms done.

3. The full report can be found at https://huc.edu/wp-content/uploads/ HUC-REPORT-OF-INVESTIGATION-11.04.21.pdf.

4. The full report can be found at https://www.ccarnet.org/wp-content/ uploads/2021/12/Alcalaw-Report-of-Investigation.pdf.

5. The full report can be found at https://urj.org/sites/default/files/2022-02/URJ_Investigation_Report.pdf.

6. Rabbi Jacob's amends video can be found at https://urj.org/blog/making-amends-message-yom-kippur-5784. The Mi Shebeirach for survivors and victims can be found at https://urj.org/sites/default/files/2023-12/ Mi_Shebayrach_for_Survivors_and_Victims.pdf.

7. The letter can be found at https://docs.google.com/document d/1IgI-BjTEYrZJV901jG5X5Yy7iWfDyoiOPjV7rBTHox4/edit?tab=t.o

8. Danya Ruttenberg, *On Repentance and Repair: Making Amends in an Unapologetic World* (Beacon Press, 2023), 84.

9. Ruttenberg, *On Repentance and Repair*, 23.

10. Ruttenberg, *On Repentance and Repair*, 36.

11. Ruttenberg, *On Repentance and Repair*, 40.

12. Dr. Guila Benchimol, personal communication with the author, September 19, 2022.

13. Ruttenberg, *On Repentance and Repair*, 41.

14. Ruttenberg, *On Repentance and Repair*, 134.

32

Leaving a Toxic Community

Ritual Moments

RABBI ROBYN ASHWORTH-STEEN

LEAVING a Jewish community following abuse, bullying, toxicity, or a betrayal of values can be an isolating, ground-shifting, and heartbreaking experience.[1] Our religious spaces can fall short of the ideals we profess. The gap between the promised land of community and the reality of fractured and toxic institutions can mean those who leave have much to process, grieve, and rage against, but without the structures that communal life offers. Finding Jewishly grounded rituals to help name and recognize the pain and potential of leaving is a necessary and urgent task. Part of the complexity of leaving a community is that sometimes it is not possible to publicly speak about the harm suffered.[2] Therefore, it is with deep gratitude that I have included anonymized testimony in this chapter from a number of people who have had to leave their community. Their honest sharing has informed this piece of writing.[3]

Emotions

"Bitterly she weeps in the night, her cheek wet with tears. . . . Judah has gone into exile because of misery and harsh oppression" (Lamentations 1:2–3).

Whether the harm suffered within a community was sexual, physical, and/or spiritual—abuse; bullying; a toxic culture; deep misalignment of values; homophobia, transphobia, ableism, racism, or so on—a complex set of emotions accompanies a separation from community. There is grief for what could have been, for what was, for relationships held, life-cycle moments marked, the regularity and familiarity of ritual and building, for the person you were. There is rage for the injustice, for the lack of accountability, at those who did not speak out, for the betrayal of the values you believed you shared. As one respondent wrote, "The worst part is when you look back to when you entered the community and realized that what you loved was already flawed and you never saw it. So, you end up not trusting yourself as well."

There is loneliness as you sit with the isolation of having to leave, losing a sense of purpose, of not being heard, of not knowing who to call in moments you would have naturally turned to the synagogue: "I miss the company of other people, human connection, the sense of belonging, knowing what's happening to other people." There is fear that you will never belong again, that the harm will continue to happen to others, that your reputation is unfairly being attacked, and that you are losing the regularity and structure of Jewish life. There is relief that you made it out and a sense of freedom.

After these initial emotions come additional ones, such as guilt and self-doubt, which can feel overwhelming and crippling. All these emotions can be heightened if the abuse and betrayal were perpetrated by the rabbi, clergy member, or respected community leaders. There are risks of moral injury (when our worldview is shaken to its core), spiritual abuse[4] (when our traditions and texts are misused and weaponized), and spiritual crises of faith and identity.

The Courage to Leave

"She took some of its fruit and ate. . . . Then the eyes of both of them were opened" (Genesis 3:6–7).

To leave a community when you have either experienced or witnessed harm is a deeply courageous move. Leaving means stepping away from all that is familiar, the structure of ritual life, and the relationships you have crafted. Leaving a community means navigating the self-doubts— "Was it me?" or "Have I got this wrong?"—and realizing that the harm is real and the structural issues are too large to ignore. To leave means to step into the unknown, perhaps by yourself, often without the harm being acknowledged or any *t'shuvah* (repentance) undertaken. This lack of acknowledgment often adds to the wounds.

While Hillel (a first-century sage) taught, "Do not separate yourself from the community" (*Pirkei Avot* 2:5), it is vital to recognize that Judaism is a religion that cares deeply about how the community acts and the necessary balancing of *chesed* (loving-kindness) and *din* (the rules of law and boundaries). For communities, this means that it is a sacred and compassionate act to ensure proper boundaries and systems of accountability are both implemented and enforced. No one should suffer or be harmed for the sake of keeping a community intact.

To be Jewish is to be part of an ongoing story of leaving and wandering, of struggle, seeking, and revelation. Our first story of leaving is that of Eve and Adam. We can now reimagine this story and, with our eyes open, look at this tale anew. Eve began to understand that the so-called Garden of Eden was no paradise. God and Adam enjoyed a close relationship, but Eve was on the margins. In one interpretation of this story, Lilith—the first woman before Eve, who had fled from Adam's unreasonable demands—came to talk to Eve in the form of a serpent to tell her of the world that existed outside of the garden.[5] Lilith encouraged Eve to reach up and eat the juicy piece of fruit from the Tree of Knowledge. Eve's eyes were opened, and she truly saw what was pleasing and harmful. She passed the fruit to Adam, and she knew, deep down, that she must leave. Once banished by God, they felt the pain of leaving as they wandered into the messy freedom before them.

Recognizing that you must leave, in order to protect yourself and to live life fully according to your values, is a courageous, ethical, *and* deeply Jewish act.

Renaming and Rediscovery

"No more shall you be called Jacob, but Israel, for you have struggled with God and human beings, and you have prevailed" (Genesis 32:29).

As Eve experienced, there is much harm and pain in leaving the known and familiar, yet there is also the potential for growth and deepening of wisdom. So too with Jacob. He spent years full of leave-takings and struggles and was subsequently renamed to honor his grown and reshaped self, forged through times of pain and discovery. We can recognize the power and strength within us and commit to finding communities where we can thrive rather than survive. Like Jacob, Sarah, Abraham, and so many of our ancestors, we are renamed through the struggle.

Rituals and Intentional Moments

"Take your time. Try not to do it alone. Trust yourself. There's no need to despair. You are still part of a community, even if you can't quite see it yet."

As this testimony teaches, there is life after leaving a community. Sometimes the moments we need to take the next step forward are not formal and planned. Sometimes it helps to have ritual moments to lean on when it feels right, even more than once. You may want to bring trusted friends along.

BLESSING OF SEPARATION FROM COMMUNITY[6]

> As I step into my Jewish tradition of leavers and wanderers, of justice seekers and brave leaders, may I find comfort through my leaving and find communities where I belong, which care and safeguard all those who join together. May I continue to make holy decisions and separate from that which harms toward that which nurtures.

> בְּרוּכָה אַתְּ שְׁכִינָה אֱלֹחֵינוּ רוּחַ הָעוֹלָם
> הַמַּבְדִּילָה בֵּין קֹדֶשׁ לְחוֹל, בֵּין אוֹר לְחֹשֶׁךְ בֵּין מָוֶת וְחַיִּים.

> *B'ruchah at Sh'chinah Eloteinu Ruach haolam,*
> *hamavdilah bein kodesh l'chol, bein or l'choshech bein mavet v'chayim.*

> Blessed are You, Shechinah (the one who accompanies us as we leave), Spirit of the universe, who distinguishes between what is holy and mundane, between light and dark, between death and life.[7]

K'RIAH: A RITUAL OF TEARING

The ritual of *k'riah* (tearing a piece of cloth) is used before a funeral to mark the visceral grief felt by mourners. In this reimagined ritual, you may wish to take a piece of cloth and make a small tear with scissors or by hand to mark the grief felt by leaving your community. You may also wish to name out loud or write on a piece of paper all that you are grieving. Once done, you may want to discard the cloth and writing or burn the items to mark letting go so that you may move forward.

MIKVEH: A RITUAL OF RENEWAL

A mikveh is a ritual bath used to mark moments of transition. Using any natural source of water, you can make three immersions, each with a different intention: for what you are leaving behind, for what you are looking forward to, and for what you wish for the present moment. You could add your own blessing or use the traditional mikveh blessing along with the *Shehecheyanu* blessing for new times.

RENAMING CEREMONY

Following in Jacob's footsteps, you may wish to add to your Hebrew name a new name that speaks to you of the person you are becoming and wish to be reminded of. With close friends and family, you may wish to say why you chose this name, ask others to add their blessings, and say the following: "Through this renaming ceremony I choose to step toward the person I am becoming and the person I aspire to be. I recognize that this name holds all the pain and beauty I have experienced until now and will support me going forward. From today I will be known as. . . . May my new name be a blessing for me and all who know me."

A SWEET RITUAL

Like Eve and Adam before you, for this ceremony take a piece of sweet fruit to mark your movement toward freedom and say whatever blessing you may need in that moment. Take your time eating the fruit, being mindful of how sensual the act is and how, in nourishing yourself, you recognize your value and beauty.

The emotions experienced when leaving a community are manifold, and the path to recovery is not linear. Go gently.

NOTES

1. The journey of reckoning with abuse in Jewish spaces is only just beginning. See Elaine Sztokman, *When Rabbis Abuse: Power, Gender, and Status in the Dynamics of Sexual Abuse in Jewish Culture* (Lioness Books, 2022); and Lisa Oakley and Justin Humphreys, *Escaping the Maze of Spiritual Abuse: Creating Healthy Christian Cultures* (SPCK, 2019).
2. Indeed, the nature of a dysfunctional and unhealthy community is "to protect itself and its reputation rather than those who have been traumatized." See Oakley and Humphreys, *Spiritual Abuse*, lix.

3. These testimonies are taken from anonymized responses to a questionnaire I sent out.
4. See Oakley and Humphreys, *Spiritual Abuse*, 31.
5. These midrashic retellings concerning Lilith can be found in these two publications: Nikki Marmery, *Lilith* (Legend Press, 2023); and Judith Plaskow, "The Coming of Lilith," in *Four Centuries of Jewish Women's Spirituality: A Sourcebook*, ed. Ellen M. Umansky and Dianne Ashton (Beacon Press, 1992), 215–16.
6. Also see Robyn Ashworth-Steen, "For When Religious Institutions Fail," in *Forms of Prayer: Prayers for the High Holydays–Yom Kippur*, 9th ed., ed. Paul Freedman and Jonathan Magonet (Movement for Reform Judaism, 2024), 711.
7. Following the Kohenet tradition of using feminine language, calling on *Shechinah*, the aspect of God associated with exile and weeping, I use the *Havdalah* ritual, which marks the distinction between the holy and unholy. See Jill Hammer and Taya Shere, *Siddur HaKohanot: A Hebrew Priestess Prayerbook* (Kohenet, 2014), 191.

33

The Unexpected Trauma of Retirement

Rabbi Daniel A. Roberts

The Eternal One spoke to Moses, saying: This is the rule for the Levites. From twenty-five years of age up they shall participate in the workforce in the service of the Tent of Meeting; but at the age of fifty they shall retire from the workforce and shall serve no more. They may assist their brother Levites at the Tent of Meeting by standing guard, but they shall perform no labor. Thus, you shall deal with the Levites in regard to their duties.

—*Numbers 8:23–26*

THE SORROW BEGAN as I sat alone in my office, with the center drawer of my desk three-quarters of the way open. I reached forward, and in the left corner was a collection of twenty-five pocket calendars—one for each year I worked—that I had carried every day in my breast pocket. I couldn't go anywhere without those little books. They were my life. I sat there staring at them, feeling very lonely. Leafing through each book, I began to wonder where all the years had gone. The calendars contained countless appointments, family and friends' birthdates, and the anniversaries of family deaths. Over those years, I hoped I had touched many people's souls, for I know they touched mine. But soon, it was going to be different. My congregants would go on with their lives, as would I.

Sitting in my almost empty office, I realized I had something in common with the Levites in the above Biblical text: retiring from the workforce. Did they feel as I did right now when notified their "godly" duties were completed, and they were to "serve no more"? Did they feel like I did, knowing their only future worth was going to be standing guard over penned-in animals while they watched the younger priests involved in the meaningful practice of preparing and offering sacrifices for God? Did they look forward to not having to do the heavy lifting of animals and being exposed to the "fire" of God, just as I anticipated not having to prepare weekly sermons and be "on call" all the time? Did their bones ache like mine after standing for an hour during service?

I wondered how the High Priest communicated the news to an individual Levite that his retirement age was approaching. Did they have some kind of ritual marking the changeover? I felt fortunate that there was going to be a "sacred moment" marking my retirement—a farewell service and social evening. My family, my friends, and those in the congregation would be present to witness this transformation. However, I began to think about how many "Levites" in my congregation may have left their careers—their life's work—with no ceremony or recognition. How many, even if they had "recognition parties," were not able to include their family and friends to witness the moment?

These questions filled my mind as I looked down at the many open boxes near my desk, all crammed with books. Which books should I keep, and which ones should I give away? I glanced at all the certificates and beautiful works of art on the walls and contemplated their futures. Each one had a special meaning to me, and I loved them.

So many tiny but overwhelming decisions put me in a state of chaos. I recalled philosopher Susanne Langer postulating that the one thing the mind cannot deal with is chaos,[1] but here I was, right in its midst. I sat in my chair by the light of the desk lamp and wanted to cry. Instead, with emotions overwhelming me, I just turned off the light, walked out of my office, and left those decisions behind.

My thoughts continued to race as I walked to my car. What was to be my new role? What was to be my future relationship with all those in the congregation? Would I see many of them again, or would we simply fade out of each other's lives? Life was going to be a *real* transition. I began to recollect the anxious moments during the summer after my senior year of high school before I left for college. Do you remember the sadness you felt watching your high school friends leave one by one for college and how worried you were about making new friends in college?

For me, retirement felt similar to that post–high school summer. Yes, I knew there would be countless new adventures in my future, but what would they be exactly? I began to deliberate whether the next adventure in my life would be as meaningful as the role I had played for the last three decades. During those thirty years, I had order in my life. Racquetball on Monday, Wednesday, and Friday mornings. Staff meetings on Tuesday mornings. Regular office hours. Friday night services. Religious school on Sunday. I had an extremely rewarding job that gave me purpose and meaning in life. I had a steady income and knew how much money I could spend monthly, but now I would have to adjust my thinking to become financially cautious. My rabbinate was my anchor, and now it was gone.

Along the way in my career, I had become certified as a thanatologist, a person who studies death, dying, and bereavement. As I rode the waves of emotion following my retirement, I recognized I was experiencing the existential grief Kenneth Doka writes about in his article "Death in Life," which I had studied during my certification process.[2] He defines existential grief as "a sense of alienation, despair, pain, or deep sorrow for a loss of meaning." I understood I needed time to grieve because retirement, for me, fit this definition.

Robert Neimeyer, a noted authority on bereavement and transition, also makes this point regarding retirement in *Lessons of Loss: A Guide to Coping*: "Unlike losses through death, there is no 'ritual' that recognizes this loss [of identity] or that provides a socially sanctioned period of grieving and recovery. If anything, social expectations run to the opposite extreme. We are expected to be relentlessly 'self-motivated' and efficient in our pursuit of a new job [that is, finding meaning is our new occupation of adjusting to retirement], at the very time that we feel most depressed, full of self-doubt, and unsure of how to proceed."[3]

I acknowledge that everyone approaches and reacts to retirement differently. Someone who hated their job may dance in joy; others may have elaborate plans for their future. Some have prepared for the moment with hobbies and interests. Other retirees are left clueless as to how they will fill the remaining moments of life. No matter what, retirement is an adjustment. Retirement calls for undoing the psychological ties that bound us to a world that provided us with security and stability, both emotionally and financially. For many, our job was the defining identity of who we were and in what category we belonged. Retirement requires us to learn to live without the daily routine we once knew. Retirement means leaving a group of people—some of whom you liked more than others—and acquiring a new cadre of friends and acquaintances with whom to socialize and interact. Retirement requires us to redefine our egos. Retirement requires us to figure out how we are going to preserve our finances, to make decisions about how and when we are going to downsize our residence, and to confront our mortality by the need to put in place legal documents regarding estate planning and end-of-life care. It means moving from days when you knew what you would be doing to waking up every morning without a set plan.

For many, like me, this disorientation is traumatic, and the transition process is made even more painful due to "disenfranchised grief," whereby those experiencing distress are not accorded a right to grieve. Ken Doka relates that ambiguous or disenfranchised grief is "the grief that persons experience when they incur a loss that is not or cannot be openly acknowledged, publicly mourned, or socially supported."[4] The business consultant William Bridges similarly argues, "Every transition involves a period of loss, then a period in the neutral zone, and then a period of rebirth. The loss that comes with retirement can be brutal.... People in the neutral zone don't yet know who the new version of themselves will be. They report feeling hollow, disoriented, empty."[5]

I felt that sense of disorientation and knew that I had to find ways to continue to be creative and find continued meaning to live. I was influenced by Abraham Joshua Heschel's essay "To Grow in Wisdom" from his book *The Insecurity of Freedom*. In it, he encourages the elderly to "attain the high values we failed to sense, the insights we have missed, [and] the wisdom we ignored."[6] From this and other readings, as well as my professional and academic work in the field of death, dying, and grief, I knew I had to—and wanted to—find a sense of significance in the new world I was about to enter, the world beyond the active rabbinate.

Going through that first year of retirement, I wished I had a cadre of like-minded people with whom I could have learned how they were handling their adjustment. I wish there were one place where I could have learned about post-retirement finances, the legal documents I would need, and how family dynamics may change. Without such a place, I began to write about my experience, having previously learned through my study of grief that journaling was a great way to handle anxiety. Among other pieces, I wrote an article for the *CCAR Journal*:

The Reform Jewish Quarterly.[7] In response, I received many emails from colleagues who shared similar emotions and trauma. My mentor, Rabbi Earl Grollman (*z"l*), a writer of countless books on death and mourning, suggested I had a book in the making. Following his advice, I coauthored a book with Dr. Michael Freidman entitled *Clergy Retirement: Every Ending a New Beginning.*[8]

Since writing the book, I have become very interested in how we can help people deal with this transitional moment. A synagogue (or a religious institution) ought to be a place in which individuals can find comraderie in entering this new stage of life, the "encore years," as some have called it. I envision a group of congregants sitting around discussing not only financial and legal issues, but also sharing community resources, volunteer opportunities, and gestures of support. I envision new friendships emerging and people turning to each other in moments of anxiety.

Not only is it important to foster welcoming, supportive community spaces, but I believe that it's also essential to create new rituals, either community-wide or private, to help people acknowledge the moment of retirement and contemplate and map out new directions for their life. We have rituals for other moments of life: birth, bet mitzvah, weddings, death, and so on. Why not retirement? I have personally written such a ritual, in which I envision family and friends gathering together and the retiree sharing possible dreams for the encore years ahead.

With as many as 11,200 Americans retiring each day,[9] the moment has arrived that we, the greater Jewish community, need both to promote the opportunity to share retirement concerns in a learning setting and to develop meaningful rituals and ceremonies to mark this sacred moment of transition.

It has been more than twenty years since I sat in that dark office gazing at those diaries. What an interesting journey from those terrifying moments to a whole new life in retirement. Besides my book *Clergy Retirement*, I have written several books on suicide and a children's book entitled *Once Upon a Kingdom*, which recounts children's stories I used to tell my youngest congregants. I never dreamed I would become an author! I have continued to grow in my encore years and have found great meaning in the activities I participate in here in the senior living community where I currently reside. I have made many wonderful new friends, which is difficult at my age, and have found that there is life after retirement—providing one is able to navigate saying goodbye to one's former life and open the doors to the next stage. Still, there is no doubt that the moment of retirement can be an interesting, traumatizing, and even revolutionary transition in anyone's life.

NOTES

1. Susanne K. Langer, *Philosophy in a New Key: A Study in the Symbolism of Reason, Rite, and Art* (Harvard University Press, 1942), 287.

2. Kenneth J. Doka, "Death in Life," in *Living with Grief: Loss in Later Life*, Kenneth J. Doka, ed. (Hospice Foundation of America, 2002), 17–33.

3. Robert Neimeyer, *Lessons of Loss: A Guide to Coping* (Memphis: Center of the Study of Loss and Transition, 2006), 34.

4. Kenneth J. Doka, *Disenfranchised Grief: Recognizing Hidden Sorrow* (Lexington Press, 1989), 4.

5. Quoted in David Brooks, "The New Old Age," *The Atlantic*, August 25, 2023, https://www.theatlantic.com/culture/archive/2023/08/career-retirement-transition-academic-programs/675085/.

6. Abraham Joshua Heschel, *The Insecurity of Freedom* (Schocken Books, 1972), 78.

7. Rabbi Daniel A. Roberts, "Mourning a Retirement: Reflections of a Thanatologist," *CCAR Journal* (Spring 2011) 49–61.

8. Daniel A. Roberts and Michael Freidman, *Clergy Retirement: Every Ending a New Beginning for Clergy, Their Family, and Congregants* (Wipf and Stock, 2017).

9. Jason J. Fichtner, "The Peak 65 Generation: Creating a New Retirement Security Framework," *Alliance for Lifetime Income*, March 30, 2021, https://www.protectedincome.org/wp-content/uploads/2021/04/ALI-White-Paper-PEAK-65-Update-4.22.21.pdf.

PART SEVEN

Trauma and Family

34

Broken Glass, Mended Heart

Healing from the Trauma of Divorce

RABBI ELIZABETH BAHAR, MAHL

D IVORCE is a part of life. For some, it is traumatic; for others, a relief. For those who experience divorce as a trauma, it can be a devastating, life-altering, challenging ordeal.

My marriage and subsequent divorce, combined with a prolonged custody battle, were traumatic. The marriage was emotionally and verbally abusive—something I did not admit to myself for a long time. Choosing to leave my marriage while working as a pulpit rabbi was a stressful decision. I assumed my congregation would judge me as a failure. How could I represent myself as a moral exemplar if I could not maintain my marriage? I was unable to see leaving my marriage as a sign of strength. I kept asking myself: How could a leader and effective communicator fail to be able to negotiate the challenges of marriage? That same question lingered as I later doubted my ability to co-parent.

As my marriage ended, I was forced to engage with the family legal system. The system is intended both to help parents who struggle to find an equitable solution when dissolving a marriage and to protect children from the stress of their parent's divorce. At the same time, it is also a capitalist system. Sometimes the lawyer's motivations in assisting their clients are for their own financial benefit rather than the best interest of the family or the children. A good lawyer can cost an exorbitant amount of money, which often leads to better judgments for their clients. However, they can file frivolous claims, causing legal bills to exceed $40,000 or more, especially if the divorce is contentious.[1] In addition, divorce is adjudicated in a court of *law* rather than *justice*, meaning that what is argued is not always about what is just, but rather what is legally permissible.

At first, my ex-spouse and I agreed on getting divorced. I thought this mutual understanding would make the process straightforward.

This was my first naive mistake. I had already been through tough times in my marriage, so I didn't expect the divorce to be any harder. I was wrong. The divorce turned out to be an emotional roller coaster that I wasn't prepared for.

Against my lawyer's advice, I entered into a settlement, forgoing child support to avoid a lengthy trial. This was another mistake.

During the course of the divorce, my youngest child was diagnosed as being on the autism spectrum and therefore would require more support than the average child. His father refused to see what physicians, therapists, and psychologists saw, so he denied that there was a need to pay for additional, medically necessary support. This was the reason for our first trip back to court. The second and third trips in front of the judge were over similar issues and resulted in a deeper understanding of our legal system. I came to understand terms such as *guardian ad litem*, *pendente lite*, and emergency return orders. I learned that a form of domestic violence utilizes the court system itself by bringing frivolous motions requiring a legal response and more lawyer fees, all with the intent of bankrupting the target of the abuse. This is the reality I was faced with.

I saw how subjective the legal system is and how limited its power is when it comes to effectively addressing emotional abuse, gaslighting, false allegations, and other similar challenges. I endured investigations about who I am and scrutiny of my parenting style, all while navigating leading a congregation, the stresses of COVID, and being a single mother.

In the end, my children's father lost all legal rights to his own children based solely on his own behavior. In hindsight, this seemed like it was the inevitable conclusion, but until we reached it, I was consumed by an overwhelming fear about the outcome of our custody battle.

As a deep thinker, I had to ask why. Why was this happening? Why is there evil? Why do some people treat others so badly and cause so much pain?

Yet, during the prolonged court cases and certainly after, I learned many things, including the possibility of post-traumatic growth (PTG) and how that applied to my life. I learned how to maintain a connection to my faith. That massive ongoing series of events has only rooted me more deeply in Judaism. I began to understand in my bones ideas from our sacred tradition that I had previously understood only intellectually. I identified with Job, who experienced tremendous loss and then felt God: "Then the Eternal replied to Job out of the tempest" (Job 38:1). I more clearly saw Aaron, who, after the death of his sons, heard God.[2] I understood Jeremiah's teaching that trusting God would nourish me (Jeremiah 17:5–8). I wish I hadn't undergone what I did. Yet, had I not, I would not have learned these deep lessons that have become so foundational and important to me now.

I will share those lessons with you with one caveat. To a great extent, people who have lived experience with certain issues acquire lessons that can only be gleaned from living with their specific types of hardship. I do not believe I would have necessarily learned these lessons any other way. I do not expect others to fully understand unless they, too, walk a similarly traumatic path.

One of these lessons from the Talmud teaches about the existence of the Mourner's Path—a special entrance through which those in mourning would enter the Temple Mount. This path existed not to separate mourners from those not in mourning, but rather to help them find a sense of community (Babylonian Talmud, *S'machot* 6a–b). Mourning causes one to feel out of step, but this dedicated path forced mourners to encounter others who were equally unmoored. I have experienced this myself. When speaking with victims of domestic violence and those going through difficult divorces where equity and even safety seem like a distant dream, there is a shared unspoken bond. We are out of step, unmoored, but together. We share the experience of being gaslighted, scrutinized, doubted, emotionally abused, exhausted, and struggling to survive. The humiliation of being deeply examined by others for who you are as a person and parent made me feel like an outsider, a pretender of being a normal and sane parent. As a rabbi, someone who is looked to for parenting and marital advice, I felt like a fraud. So despite the limitations of walking through a door that is not entirely one's own, I share the lessons and growth that resulted from the trauma of my divorce.

From the challenging marriage, the divorce, and the subsequent custody battle, I learned four big lessons. The first lesson was about forgiveness.

A deep comprehension of forgiveness comes from experiencing great wrongs and working through every facet of releasing resentment. I walked a path of deeply understanding the lesson of forgiveness by forgiving myself for marrying my former spouse. I had to forgive myself for looking for somebody else to be the solution to my inner pain. I had to forgive myself for dreaming of a knight on a white horse stepping in to rescue me. My inner pain stems from my own fears of being unloved and unlovable. I had to recognize that my fear of being abandoned exists because as a child I was bullied and experienced rejection. I needed to uncover the wounds that I brought into my marriage so I could finally heal from them. I also had to struggle with forgiveness, since it is one of those things that is easy to say and hard to do. In forgiving myself, I had to grasp that love is not simply an emotion we feel, but is what we do. It is expressed in how we treat ourselves and others. I have moments when anger and resentment still well up inside me. But forgiving myself allowed me to also forgive my former spouse.

For anyone going through a similar experience, the path to forgiveness—of oneself and others—is crucial but challenging. It requires deep self-reflection and a willingness to let go of pain and resentment. We can only do better when we know better. I had to learn that the need for forgiveness and letting go of carrying anger and pain is the equivalent of constantly carrying a lump of hot coal and then putting it down. Carrying that hot coal drains us and increases the burden of pain. We are the only ones who are being burned by it. Putting it down frees us from the pain of holding on to the anger so tightly.

The second lesson I learned was a soul lesson, as I sought to find meaning in my excruciating experience. I formed a narrative that life is about learning lessons on a soul level, and everything we experience is meant to teach us something.

I believe that humanity's purpose is to learn from and experience life. To do that, we place other human beings in roles in our lives to help us enact and reenact stories that we tell ourselves or to help us heal our wounds. We continuously relive those stories until we have understood the lessons we need to learn. For example, we might experience abandonment repeatedly, each time in a more significant and painful way, until we learn not to abandon ourselves. Similarly, we may face situations requiring forgiveness until we understand the need to let go. Each person will need to learn lessons on a soul level in their own way.

This belief is based on my understanding of a midrash found in the Talmud:

> Rabbi Simlai delivered the following discourse: What does an embryo resemble when it is in the bowels of its mother? Folded writing tablets. . . . A light burns above its head and it looks and sees from one end of the world to the other. . . . And there is no time in which a person enjoys greater happiness than in those days. . . . It is also taught all the Torah from beginning to end. . . . As soon as it sees the light, an angel approaches, slaps it on its mouth and causes it to forget all the Torah completely. (Babylonian Talmud, *Nidah* 30b)[3]

As fetuses, we are illuminated by the light of knowledge and Torah. At birth, an angel metaphorically "slaps" this knowledge out of us, leaving only the philtrum under our noses as a reminder of this encounter. Throughout life, we gradually relearn and deepen our understanding of these truths. This process of recalling and relearning allows us to find redemption and growth, even through our most challenging experiences. The knowledge that we need to learn is stored in the recesses of our memories, but only partly. As we go through life, we relearn what once was lost. As we study or live, we are both recalling something and learning it on a deeper level. Understanding and embracing these lessons allow us to find redemption and growth, even through our most challenging experiences.

The third lesson I learned was about healing, a process that occurs not in isolation but rather in relationships.

I deeply believe in the truth taught by Rabbi Lawrence Kushner in his poem "Jigsaw," which teaches that "no one has within themselves all the pieces to their puzzle. . . . Everyone carries with them at least one and probably many pieces to someone else's puzzle."[4] I understand this to mean that we are all born with some knowledge that we need and some knowledge that seems extraneous but is necessary for us to share with someone else. We do not know how needed that knowledge is until someone else receives it. As such, we are deeply enmeshed with one another. Sometimes giving and receiving these puzzle pieces can cause hurt; sometimes, though, the sharing leads to healing.

These life lessons of forgiveness, understanding the soul-reason for my marriage, increased compassion, and self-reliance helped me fully mourn the loss of my marriage and explain why the trauma occurred.

The lengthy, drawn-out custody battle—including over $100,000 in debt from legal bills and the fear of losing my children—provided the opportunity for my fourth, deep lesson—post-traumatic growth.

PTG differs from resiliency or simply returning to the daily life that existed before the trauma. PTG is a direct and beneficial consequence of trauma, allowing someone to reach heights otherwise impossible. It is not shrinking from the events, but flourishing in its aftermath. We read in the Book of Exodus, "But the more they were oppressed, the more they increased and spread out, so that the [Egyptians] came to dread the Israelites" (Exodus 1:12). As the Israelites suffered in Egypt, they were forced into a diminished position, but they decided to grow, to receive blessings. Life placed them into a crucible, and instead of being crushed, they grew stronger and unbroken.

Most people who walk the path of PTG will eventually learn to accept what life presents.

In the words of Rabbi Harold Kushner, who wrote about the loss of his son and the resulting theological reckoning in his famous book *When Bad Things Happen to Good People*:

> I am a more sensitive person, a more effective pastor, a more sympathetic counselor because of Aaron's life and death than I would ever have been without it. And I would give up all of those gains in a second if I could have my son back. If I could choose, I would forgo all the spiritual growth and depth which has come my way because of our experiences, and be what I was fifteen years ago, an average rabbi, an indifferent counselor, helping some people and unable to help others, and the father of a bright, happy boy. But I cannot choose.[5]

I also could not choose. So, I walked and at times stumbled the path of PTG. I realized that I am not alone, as God is everywhere, even though I felt deep loneliness throughout the entire marriage, divorce, and custody battle. When I was able to sit in silence, I felt connected to God. My path reinforced the knowledge that I could meet my own needs without an unhealthy dependence on someone else and that God can send angels in the form of kind, generous people to help me.[6]

Today, I am pulling myself slowly out of debt. My children are mourning the regular presence of their father, who can visit them only with court supervision. Still, we breathe freely in peace and quiet for the first time in six years.

I no longer need to choose between my congregation and my children. As a result of everything that I experienced, my life with my children will always come first. There will always be things to do, tasks to accomplish, and board meetings to attend, but my time with them is priceless. I could only have come to that realization and release after enduring everything that happened. Now, the simple joy of a family game night gives me a sense of immense gratitude.

I can choose to focus on my suffering, recognizing that many of the circumstances that I walked through were beyond my control. But instead, I choose to focus on the lessons I learned and my own inner narrative. I can finally cherish the wound and live an authentic, complete life.

NOTES

1. Chauncey Crail, "How Much Does a Divorce Cost in 2025?," *Forbes Advisor Online*, July 29, 2022, https://www.forbes.com/advisor/legal/divorce/how-much-does-divorce-cost/.
2. Rashi on Leviticus 10:3.
3. This translation is from the William Davidson digital edition of the *Koren Talmud*, with commentary by Rabbi Adin Even-Israel Steinsaltz (Koren Publishers), found on Sefaria (sefaria.org).
4. Rabbi Lawrence Kushner, *Honey from the Rock: Visions of Jewish Mystical Renewal* (Jewish Lights Publishing, 1992), 69–70.
5. Rabbi Harold S. Kushner, *When Bad Things Happen to Good People* (Anchor Books, 1981), 133–34.
6. "And so we understand that ordinary people are messengers of the Most High. They go about their tasks in holy anonymity, often, even unknown to themselves. Yet, if they had not been there, if they had not said what they said or did what they did, it would not be the way it is now. We would not be the way we are now. Never forget that you, too, yourself may be a messenger. Perhaps even one whose errand extends over several lifetimes." Lawrence Kushner, *Honey from the Rock*, 74. Also quoted in *Mishkan T'Filah: A Reform Siddur* (CCAR Press, 2007), 143.

35

Conceiving Hope

Navigating Infertility in the Jewish Community

Rabbi Jen Gubitz

"WE HAVEN'T SEEN YOU IN A WHILE," I write to her in a quick email. It's 2011 and I'm a rabbinical student leading High Holy Days services for Brooklyn Jews, a project of Congregation Beth Elohim in Park Slope, Brooklyn.

"I read in your High Holy Day registration," my email continues, "that you had a tough year. I hope you're doing okay."

Her name is also Jen, and I really mean it when I express that sentiment about her well-being. However, fifteen years later, I realize I probably didn't actually know what "okay" meant.

"I couldn't bear to see the strollers in the lobby," she emails back. "The thought of watching new families stand up in front of the congregation for a blessing was too much for me. It still makes me cry just to think about it."

The blessing she was referring to was an invitation during the Rosh HaShanah Torah service to those who had welcomed a new child in the past year. It was among the many life-cycle moments we sought to celebrate during Rosh HaShanah, a moment in our Jewish calendar pregnant with purpose, renewal, and rebirth. It was a loud and joyful moment as parents and new babies came up for a cacophony of Hebrew blessings and baby babbling. But it was not joyful for everyone, I soon came to learn.

As a twenty-seven-year-old rabbinical student, I'd never thought about strollers in the synagogue lobby as a potential emotional trigger. The only exposure I'd had to babies and motherhood was when Sara, my closest friend in rabbinical school at Hebrew Union College–Jewish Institute of Religion, gave birth to the most magnificent creature I'd ever met. I was so excited for her when she showed me the positive pregnancy test in our rabbinical school bathroom one morning after Bible class. I sat next to her in classes the entire year as she lovingly incubated her child until the baby arrived in October of our third year of school. To celebrate, I selected a handmade baby blanket with the baby's Hebrew and English names knitted into it, a gift I would send forty-six more times to celebrate my loved ones welcoming their new babies.

But in 2011, my congregant Jen taught me about a different perspective. I was grateful she was willing to share her fertility journey with me (and for her permission to share about it in this piece); it was one of sorrow and of great grief as she longed for a child.

"It's been devastating, life-changing, disorienting. . . . Infertility . . . seems to ruin pretty much everything in your life in one way or another. But, we are surviving, coping, and have lots and lots and lots of amazing support from family, friends, therapists, doctors. I've found a way to cope in nearly all parts of my life, but not yet with Judaism."

I'd always believed Judaism had the capacity to hold us in our greatest joys and deepest sorrows. But was that actually true? Could I, as a spiritual guide and almost rabbi, help this community member find ways for Judaism to support her throughout her isolation and grief?

Perhaps comfort lay in the ancient stories of the Jewish people. Our Torah is full of Biblical matriarchs who are barren. Abraham's wife Sarah (Genesis 11:30), Isaac's wife Rebekah (Genesis 25:21), and Jacob's wife Rachel (Genesis 29:31) all struggle to conceive children. Biblical scholar Robert Alter refers to these stories as "annunciation scenes," literary devices that foreshadow the birth of an important patriarch.[1] Their barrenness only shifts when God intervenes—hearing their cries, remembering their struggle—and opens their wombs.[2] From each of their great sorrows, a great patriarch is born: Sarah bears Isaac, Rebekah bears Jacob, and Rachel bears Joseph. It seems that the matriarchs' stories are wrapped up in a tidy bow as their wombs determine the next chapter in the story of the Jewish people. But what of their sorrow? And for a modern person struggling with infertility, would these stories actually resonate or offer comfort?

It wasn't until September 2021 that I personally understood the grief of my long-ago congregant Jen, the plight of our barren Biblical matriarchs, and the experiences of the many young adults struggling with infertility whom I've served as a rabbi.

That Rosh HaShanah, my husband and I were logged into Zoom services at our shul, Temple Beth Zion in Brookline, Massachusetts. We stayed home because we were in the middle of our second IVF egg retrieval cycle. While being exposed to Jewish community and High Holy Day prayer may have been uplifting after a year of pandemic isolation, exposure to or diagnosis of COVID-19 would cancel the two-week cycle of twice daily hormonal injections meant to stimulate my ovaries into over-producing eggs.

As a rabbi, I deeply understood the themes—creation, renewal, rebirth, sweetness, and joy—of the High Holy Day season. I knew quite well the Rosh HaShanah haftarah reading from the prophetic Book of Samuel about Hannah sitting in the Temple in Shiloh, praying for God to give her a child.[3] And I understood viscerally, for the first time, why the ancient Hannah was murmuring, longing, whispering, begging, praying for a child—because we were too. Throughout that day, I livestreamed Rosh HaShanah services across the country in search of comfort and connection. But instead, my body was bloated, and we felt socially isolated. The ancient stories of the Jewish people were grating to hear, and I turned on Shark Tank reruns when the story of Hannah was read. It was too much to bear. It seemed that the God who remembered Sarah, Rebekah, Rachel, and Hannah did not remember me. Although that IVF cycle was considered successful and yielded three genetically normal embryos, the sweetness of that New Year—and several Jewish New Years to come—eluded us.

Many people have a growing awareness of infertility, but the statistics are staggering. According to the World Health Organization, one in six couples struggle with infertility, "a disease of the male or female reproductive system defined by the failure to achieve a pregnancy after 12 months or more of regular unprotected sexual intercourse."[4] By the time my husband and I met when we were thirty-five years old, I was already in the medical category of "advanced maternal age." Having counseled and supported so many individuals and couples struggling to build their families, I anticipated that we might encounter some fertility challenges, but we had no idea to what extent. Ultimately, over the course of nearly four years, I endured four IVF cycles, three uterine surgeries, multiple diagnostic tests, and had pumped my body full of hormones—the impact of which I still feel today. At the end of that entire process, I was advised that it was not medically safe for me to try to carry a pregnancy.

Even with decent health insurance coverage, the financial toll was tremendous; the emotional toll was even greater. Through my work as the founder of Modern Jewish Couples,[5] a Jewish learning project that supports couples on the pathway to marriage and beyond, I officiated thirty weddings and helped families welcome fifteen new babies. I continued to send those personalized Hebrew baby blankets to my friends who were welcoming new children. I did not wish our infertility journey on anyone, and when I was wearing my professional hat, I also knew that their joy and my personal sorrow could coexist. But many friends and many congregants had already had at least two children by the time we found out that surrogacy or adoption was our best pathway to building our family. While it was not easy to watch others celebrate something I wanted so desperately, I tried to let their joy wash over me. As I wrote in a *Romper* article in May of 2022, "Each time, I expect it and it still catches me off guard as grandparents' eyes gleam with pride and brim with emotion; as exhausted parents yawn and smile, grateful for the health of their new child; as baby sleeps through this first life ritual, transformation tucked away into their onesie and their soul."[6] Over time, I realized I could choose resentment or I could let these moments help me continue to conceive hope that we would one day celebrate too.

My husband and I were lucky to have one another, our families, and closest friends for support. But our social circles shrank as some friends with children began to build their lives around nap schedules and playground meetups, until gradually they stopped spending time with us. As the years of our marriage went by, I would notice acquaintances, community members, colleagues, and congregants greeting me with a full body scan. "Is she pregnant yet?" I sensed them wondering. People would casually ask us, "Do you have kids?" or "Do you want kids?" Though never asked with poor intentions, these questions added insult to injury to my already bruised body and soul.

My main source of meaningful comfort and connection was spending time with others who had experienced challenging fertility journeys, who understood what it was like to wait for a fertility clinic to call you back with test results, who also spent hours a day fighting with their insurance companies, who had tricks for tolerating painful injections, who had grieved pregnancy loss, or who would socialize with us outside even on cold New England winter days so we could avoid COVID exposure. There were also many friends and loved ones who may not have experienced infertility but who would say to me, "Can I ask you how things are going?" They helped restore my agency when I felt powerless. I could say "no" if I didn't want to talk about how things were going, and I could say "yes" if I was ready to share.

I recently reflected back on my 2011 email exchange with my Brooklyn Jews congregant Jen. In those emails, I had suggested a number of rituals and readings that might bring her comfort, like the stories of the matriarchs and the Rosh HaShanah reading about Hannah. I reminded her that she was not alone in the Jewish community and offered to go with her to the mikveh as a way to pursue a measure of healing. I let her know that we would still be offering blessings for new children and growing families on Rosh HaShanah because it's important for Jewish communities to celebrate the joys experienced by many, even while others may grieve. However, because of what Jen taught us, we would also offer a blessing "for the Hannahs among us"—all those yearning to create and birth someone or something into the world:

> *Mi Shebeirach imoteinu, Sarah, Rivkah, Rachel v' Chanah . . .*
> May the One who blessed our foremothers,
> Sarah, Rebekah, Rachel, and Hannah,
> when they each sought You in their longing for a child,
> bless those and answer those who call out to You now.
> Continue to be a source of life
> and a source of hope for all who seek You.
> For all who yearn to be a parent,
> may the coming year be one of healing and vitality,
> deliverance and consolation,
> fruitfulness and joy,
> goodness and profound blessing.[7]

But most of all, I continued to check in with Jen to see how she was doing, was very mindful about the types of questions I asked, and let her decide when and what she wanted to share with me. I'm not sure if the Jewish sources I shared with her were a source of comfort or if the act of reaching out to her was more important.

Many months later, Jen and I met at the West Side Mikvah in Manhattan so she could immerse in the ritual waters to mark the transition to building her family through adoption. While not all fertility journeys result in a child, I was elated to receive an email later that year with the subject line "Our Family." In December 2012, Jen and her then-husband Josh welcomed a new baby girl into the world through adoption. They named her Hannah.

When I was officiating a wedding a few years back, the couple had just signed their *ketubah* when a loving grandfather chimed in: "Rabbi, I didn't hear anything in that *ketubah* about having grandchildren as soon as possible."

While I quickly and humorously responded, "Grandpa, we need to focus on one life-cycle transformation at a time," his comment and other frequent jokes like that at weddings stayed with me. His comment was well-meaning and imbued with hope, but I wondered who else in the room might feel its unintended sting.

Much of the reason the Jewish community exists today is because of a deep focus on passing on Jewish tradition, ritual, stories, and memory to future generations. But expecting or assuming that everyone will be able to or even *want* to physically birth a child into the world creates barriers and limitations on who might feel actively included in the Jewish community.

In my work with Modern Jewish Couples, we never assume that anyone is planning to birth children into the world or even want to become parents at all. Instead, we ask couples, "How do you define family? And what do you hope your family will look like in five or ten years? Is it a community of friends, furry animals, tiny humans, or something else?" For those interested in having children, we talk about genetic testing, fertility, and pathways to family building—including the various resources in the Jewish community that support those on fertility journeys.[8]

How we talk about family, children, fertility, and infertility can have a deep impact on our loved ones and our broader Jewish community. Instead of asking people if they have kids, we can ask, "Who's in your family?" And when we only communally honor those who have experienced a celebration of the family life cycle like marriage or birth, we limit our opportunities to honor the joys and sorrows of being human for those whose life trajectories diverge from the traditional understandings of Jewish continuity.

In our ancient Jewish stories, we learn that God remembers Sarah, Rebekah, Rachel, and Hannah, and they each give birth to important patriarchs who carry forward the story of the Jewish people. There are so many places to turn to in Jewish tradition for comfort in difficult moments, whether they are these stories of the matriarchs, contemporary writing, rituals for aspects of fertility treatment, comforting music, or Jewish support groups. There are also many customs related to fertility—mikveh ritual bath immersions or eating the *pitom* (tip) of an etrog at the end of Sukkot.[9] What is helpful, however, is unique for every person; one can try out different modalities to see if it helps them, knowing that there is always another pathway to explore. Although those Jewish stories I offered my congregant were never quite a balm for my soul, I understand deeply the power of being apart from and part of the collective Jewish narrative. I hope this understanding will continue to help me be a better friend and rabbi.

The ritual that got me through our grief was Jewish music. We listened on repeat to songs that prayed for healing, songs that spoke to the narrowness of being human, and songs that imagined God as a healer of the brokenhearted. I created a Spotify playlist to share with others who might be seeking solace too. Alongside music, speaking and writing about our experiences publicly to reduce the stigma of infertility helped me transform my grief into something that felt useful and reclaim some of my personal agency in a powerless time.

And while not all fertility journeys get tied up in a bow, our story finally had a joyful outcome too. I am still astonished by the generosity of mind, body, and spirit we experienced when my dear friend from rabbinical school—Rabbi Jill Avrin—offered to be our gestational carrier. After months of extensive medical, legal, financial, and patient navigation, one of those little embryos created during that lonely Rosh HaShanah in 2021 was transferred to Jill's uterus in late July of 2023. We found out the embryo transfer was successful and that Jill was pregnant on Tu B'Av, the Jewish day of love. On Friday, March 22, 2024—shortly before the festival of Purim—our son, Ori Shir, entered the world. In accordance with tradition, we selected the initials of his name to honor loved ones in our families. Our fertility journey added further depth. His middle name, Shir, "song," was for the music that brought us such comfort. We named him Ori, "my light," because his existence brings us light after so many dark years.

And that dear friend from rabbinical school, Sara, sent us a soft, purple blanket personalized with musical notes and Ori Shir's name written in Hebrew and English letters, knitting together a very long journey of sorrow and hope.

NOTES

1. Robert Alter, *The Art of Biblical Narrative* (Basic Books, 1981), 47–62.
2. After years of barrenness, God remembers Sarah (Genesis 21:1), and she bears Isaac. As an adult, Isaac pleads to God (Genesis 25:21) on behalf of his wife Rebekah, and she conceives and bears their twin sons, Jacob and Esau. Jacob eventually weds both Leah and her sister Rachel. As Leah and their handmaidens bear child upon child, Rachel remains barren until God eventually also remembers her, hearing her sorrows and opening her womb to give birth to Joseph (Genesis 30:22).
3. The haftarah prophetic reading for Rosh HaShanah comes from the Book of I Samuel. We encounter Hannah sitting in the Temple in Shiloh praying to God for a child. The priest Eli, misunderstanding her private prayer for drunkenness, rebukes her until she explains she is praying for a child. Eli blesses her prayers and in time, God remembers Hannah (I Samuel 1:19). She gives birth to Samuel, who becomes a judge, priest, and prophet who anoints Saul and David as kings of Israel.
4. World Health Organization, "Infertility," May 22, 2024, https://www.who.int/news-room/fact-sheets/detail/infertility.
5. To learn more, visit www.modernjewishcouples.com.
6. Rabbi Jen Gubitz, "A Mother's Day Garden of Grief," *Romper*, May 6, 2022, https://www.romper.com/pregnancy/unexplained-infertility-mothers-day.
7. Rabbi Elana Perry, "Mi Shebeirach," Hasidah, https://www.hasidah.org/wp-content/uploads/2017/03/Prayers-and-Readings-Page.pdf. Used by permission.
8. Two examples of Jewish organizations conducting such work are I Was Supposed to Have a Baby and the Jewish Fertility Foundation.

9. There are many connections between an *etrog* and fertility. One folk custom holds that a person in labor could ease labor pains by sleeping with the *pitom* (tip) under the pillow. Another advises eating a *pitom* to assist with fertility.

36

Im Yirtzeh HaShem
Rebuilding a Shattered Theology After Stillbirth

RABBI KAREN GLAZER PEROLMAN

I DIDN'T GROW UP with Jewish superstitions. No salt thrown over my shoulder or Yiddish aphorisms muttered by a grandparent. As a born-and-raised Reform Jew, I was first raised in and then gravitated toward the rational parts of religion. I marched for social justice issues, attended Shabbat services, and planned youth group events. I knew I believed, but I didn't connect much with God except to utter a prayer when I knew I didn't study enough for a test or wanted someone at camp to ask me to the end-of-summer dance.

My theology began to develop during rabbinical school. I came to understand that just as I learned Torah and life cycles, I would need to also find a way to think about God beyond the spiritual vending machine I had personalized. Through study and prayer and a deepening of my personal spirituality, I came to understand a divine presence in my life: one that was both limited and expansive, all-good but not all-powerful, and one that I could connect with in my most difficult moments.

This emerging theological understanding came into focus during my summer chaplaincy training, specifically during a workshop on postnatal loss. The nurse who specialized in working with families after the loss of a pregnancy or death of an infant made it clear that the role of a chaplain, especially one who served as a congregational clergyperson, would be helping people make sense of their losses and that pregnancy and baby loss would be among the most difficult, but also most important, losses. "Don't ever assume," she said unemotionally and firmly. "Pregnancy does not always mean a baby." She sternly warned us against ever remarking on what might look like a pregnant belly or asking questions more appropriate for a friend than a rabbi.

Those lessons served me well when, a few years later, a woman in my congregation—a young mom of two, with one on the way—called me in hysterics. At her twenty-week anatomy scan, they found out that due to a genetic abnormality, the baby could not live outside the womb. She was devastated, and her questions felt impossible to answer: Why was this happening? Did she somehow deserve it? Was this a punishment or a sign? I didn't have any answers. I didn't know if my job was to defend God's "plan" or to be angry at God on her behalf. But eighteen months later, I praised God when I named her new baby daughter on a beautiful summer morning.

Over time, I learned how many congregants and friends had difficult roads to parenthood and how these struggles caused them to reevaluate their relationship with God. One person asked me to bless a red string she would wear during her fertility treatments. Another took on a new Hebrew name, hoping to change her "divine luck." Others dove into studying the matriarchs and Biblical women who had experienced infertility. One such story is that of Hannah, which is traditionally read as the haftarah, the prophetic reading, on Rosh HaShanah. Hannah is so outwardly bereft from her barrenness that the High Priest, Eli, mistakes her for being intoxicated. But her story has a happy ending: She is granted a child, whom she names Samuel. Hannah's story of conception and birth is a redemptive pairing with the themes of renewal and rebirth that are at the core of the Jewish High Holy Day season.

My story also seemed to be heading toward a happy ending. During my first decade as a rabbi, I experienced a personal whirlwind: an engagement, wedding, short first marriage, divorce, healing, and finally meeting someone with whom I was ready to build a family. We both were of "advanced maternal age," so we didn't have much time to waste; we chose a sperm donor and made embryos. Eight weeks after my thirty-ninth birthday, I was pregnant.

Though I had never been superstitious, I found myself not taking anything for granted. I wasn't sure exactly why, but I brushed off the wishes of *mazal tov* (congratulations) and mentally corrected them, saying to myself *b'shaah tovah* (may it be at a good time)—a traditional Jewish salutation for pregnancy. This phrase indicates the uncertainty of pregnancy and the hope that the fetus grows into a living baby. I also dutifully wrote IY"H, the abbreviation for *im yirtzeh HaShem* (if God wills it), next to each doctor's appointment and future milestone in my calendar, as if to prove that it was all beyond my control. These rituals became a way I connected with the divine partnership of conception and birth. I was really nervous. I calmed my anxiety by hoping that if I just acknowledged God's part in the life growing inside me, I would be protected from all the bad things I knew were possible. And after seven months of ordinary appointments, I began to relax and joyfully expect what I was expecting.

A few weeks later, the situation quickly changed. At thirty-three weeks and six days pregnant, I went into labor in the middle of the night. Our daughter, Leo Pearl, was stillborn at 7:17 a.m. on November 10, 2021. Unbeknownst to me, I had been experiencing severe preeclampsia and needed immediate medical attention. It was a harrowing few hours, but once I was stable, the nurses asked if we wanted to speak to a member of the clergy. Indeed, half the people in and out of our room those first twenty-four hours were rabbis and cantors—my colleagues and friends who helped us begin to plan a funeral and brought company and comfort.

But once they all left, my wife and I were left with the silence of an empty room. Our daughter lay in the newborn warming tray. We held her and took pictures, trying to somehow connect with her lifeless body. Until that morning, "stillbirth" was not a word that I had ever remembered saying, but in the back of my mind, it awoke a verse from the Torah I had studied in rabbinical school.

When Aaron and Miriam gossip about their brother Moses, Miriam is punished with *tzaraat*, a scaly affliction. This physical ailment must have been very scary and upsetting to witness, for Aaron says to his brother, "Let her [Miriam] not be like a stillbirth which emerges from its mother's womb with half its flesh eaten away!" (Numbers 12:12).[1] The imagery was too much. It felt cruel that tradition used my daughter's permanent and eternal state as a physical insult, a condition brought upon as punishment. In the dark of the hospital room, I tried to find some light in the commentary to comfort me or some reading of the text that would soften the blow.

No ancient or modern commentary did much to explain the text's use of the word "stillbirth" to describe Miriam's skin separating from her body. But this ailment causes the first recorded spontaneous prayer in the Torah: "So Moses cried out to the Eternal, saying, 'O God, pray heal her!'" (Numbers 12:13). I also wanted to cry out to be healed, but between the lifesaving medications pumping into my veins and having not slept in more than twenty-four hours, my spiritual crisis began to unfurl. Through my tears, I cursed God for causing me so much pain, for not ensuring my medical team caught my complications, and for the insensitivity of those who misgendered our daughter for her name or, even worse, referred to her as a "fetal demise." I hated that after I was released from the hospital I would have to bury my daughter and utter cruel words of praise to our Creator.

I'm not sure if it was spiritual muscle memory or a deep desire to make my daughter's funeral beautiful, but despite my crisis of faith, I leaned into the mourning rituals. Her burial was held as soon as possible, we gave her a Hebrew name, and our bereaved circle of friends filled her grave with earth. Words I had said hundreds of times as a funeral officiant somehow comforted me as a mourner. My rabbinic colleague shared an interpretive translation of Psalm 23:

> Adonai is now the shepherd of this child:
> God, allow her to lie down,
> Allow her to play in green pastures,
> Allow her to feel the love of her parents and family,
> Lead her and hold her and give her warmth and comfort.
> Now we stand in the valley of dark, evil shadows;
> > help us not to be afraid.
> Comfort and support us with Your rod and staff.
> Provide for us and bolster us when the world seems too much to bear.
> God, we pray—allow the memory of goodness, mercy, and hope
> > to remain with us forever.[2]

In the months after Leo's stillbirth, my theological questions grew painful and unanswerable: Did my daughter have a soul? Was she with my father-in-law, my *bubbe*, my friend who died young from cancer? Was this Leo's predestined fate? Why did this terrible thing happen to me? How was I to continue to live in a world without my baby?

I returned to my rabbinic work newly awakened to the theological quandary that was now my life. How was I to teach about a God who had failed me so spectacularly? Or praise a God who gave someone a living baby and me a dead one? Or sit with a struggling bar mitzvah student who brazenly told me that he didn't believe in God? (Me neither!) I felt perpetually anxious and jumpy as well as theologically, professionally, and personally lost. I found myself most at home with mourners—at the funeral home and cemetery, gathering in minyan during shivah, and even during my first year of mourning as I did double duty leading *Kaddish* as a rabbi and saying *Kaddish* as a grieving parent.[3]

The landscape of grief literature is ever expanding as grief is accepted as a normal part of life. Though there is much written, the Jewish grief space is limited. I reread Viktor Frankl's work and Rabbi Harold Kushner's *When Bad Things Happen to Good People*. In the secular realm, books like *It's OK That You're Not OK*, *Bearing the Unbearable*, *The Year of Magical Thinking*, and *The Grieving Brain* anchored me. When I couldn't be comforted by God, God's creatures gave me the greatest comfort.

Ten months after Leo's stillbirth, we dedicated her headstone and unveiled it, marking a permanent place for her and for us to be with her. Her stone reads, *Adonai Lah V'Lo Nira*, a reinterpretation of the last line of *Adon Olam*. Rather than "God is with me, I will not fear," the translation on her stone reads, "God is with her, we will not fear." Despite my doubts, that was my theological truth. I was desperately sad. I missed my daughter and the mother I wanted to be for her. I longed for the innocence of that first positive pregnancy test and the whooshing fetal heartbeat. I was jealous of those who had the privilege of never knowing my pain. But I was not afraid. I didn't worry that Leo was in pain or not cared for. I did not fear that I hadn't taken care of her while she was in my care. That shift allowed me to pursue another pregnancy. When we visited Leo's grave on her first *yahrzeit*, I was ten weeks pregnant with her little sister Eloise, *baruch HaShem* (praise God), born alive and healthy in May of 2023.

My second pregnancy was also filled with superstitions, but I performed them with my eyes wide open. I knew the terrible things that were possible, and I held on to every milestone we reached. I knew there was no amount of praying or repetitive quirks that would change the outcome. There was no moment when I relaxed. Instead, I prayed for the strength to withstand the unknowable nature of life and death.

Though the stillbirth of my daughter remains a cavernous and complex pain that has fundamentally altered the direction and meaning of my life, I am simultaneously dismayed and comforted knowing that I am not alone in this pain. An unknowable number of people have lost babies in pregnancy and at birth; it is an unfairly common pregnancy outcome, especially for women of color, LGBTQ individuals, and others who are discriminated against by our health-care system. The statistics are grim: twenty-one thousand babies each year die before their due dates, and 1 out of 175 pregnancies will end with parents leaving the hospital with broken hearts and empty arms.[4]

I used to think that my theology was broken. There is no magic glue when something is simultaneously so strong and so fragile, but over time I have found a way to build something new. It is still fragile, but with a surprising resilience. Like the glass broken at a wedding, the shattering of my pre-grief theology has opened the door for something new. It is a newness I wish I didn't know, but one that is the second half of my soul's unique curriculum in this world.

Each time I officiate at a funeral I am struck again by the words of Psalm 23, especially its middle verse. At Leo's funeral, the interpretation was read: "Now we stand in the valley of dark, evil shadows; help us not to be afraid."[5] In repeating its ancient, meditative words, I have come to love how this verse transitions the psalm from third to first person. We move from speaking *about* God to speaking *to* God. And in speaking directly with our Creator, we can vocalize our deepest fears—that we will be left alone to bear the burden of our grief.

Herbert Kretzmer, the English lyricist, wrote the oft-quoted lyrics from *Les Miserables*, "To love another person is to see the face of God." For me, seeing my living daughter's face helped me find a love for the God that I wrestle intensely with, but whose presence I also seek. When I look into Eloise's eyes, I almost imagine that I can see into Leo's eyes and perhaps even into some kind of divine portal. In that space I see all the babies born, all those lost before birth, and all those yet to be. And I can see the shadow of a God who has walked with me this far and who, *im yirtzeh HaShem*, will walk with me, and all of us, for all the days to come.

NOTES

1. Biblical translations are from *The JPS Tanakh: Gender-Sensitive Edition* (Jewish Publication Society, 2023), found on Sefaria (sefaria.org).

2. Translation by Rabbi Jim Egolf, DMin, DDiv, ACPE certified educator. Used by permission. Found in *L'chol Z'man V'eit: For Sacred Moments* (CCAR Press, 2015), 60.

3. The *Kaddish*, also known as *Kaddish Yatom* or the Mourner's Kaddish, is a prayer focused on God's greatness and goodness and is recited daily for eleven montha after a loss and on the anniversary of a loss.

4. "Data and Statistics on Stillbirth," US Centers for Disease Control and Prevention, last modified May 15, 2024, https://www.cdc.gov/stillbirth/data-research/index.html.

5. Psalm 23 is often translated as "Though I walk through the valley of the shadow of death, I will fear no evil, for You are with me."

37

Seeking Solace

Faith After My Father's Suicide

DEBORAH L. GREENE

MY FATHER, Lowell Herman, *z"l*, died by suicide on April 20, 2015. The news of his death left me with a definitive and abrupt break in my life. There was the me that I was before losing him and the me I became in the aftermath. Mourning my father's death was complicated. At one of the first support groups that I attended, a fellow survivor of suicide loss shared that I would have to learn to live with the knowledge that the father I loved had taken the life of the father I loved. Grappling with this unimaginable moral complexity, I found myself searching for clues, missed signs, anything that would help me to answer the haunting question of *why*. This process, I came to understand, was the "psychological autopsy" journey that most survivors of suicide loss embark upon. I was traumatized and lost, trying to navigate the valley of shadows without a compass. I turned to my faith, searching for sources of comfort, prayers, anything that would speak to the loss of a loved one by suicide. Prior to his death, my relationship to Jewish text and liturgy was tenuous at best, but the chasm grew deeper and wider after I lost him.

My search for solace came up empty, except for the myriad of articles I found expanding on the now archaic belief that suicide was once a sin in Judaism. The fact I could not find anything to ease my pain was the first crack in the foundation of my faith. At a time when I most needed to find grounding, there was none. Unable to see my pain reflected anywhere in the lexicon of my faith or to find reverence for the way my father had died, even the tenuous grasp that tethered me to my Jewish community weakened.

I wanted to observe the tradition of saying *Kaddish* at shul for my father.[1] I can't explain why that felt important to me, but it did. Yet the liturgy that permeated services—prayers to an all-powerful God—made even the small act of trying to honor my father fraught with pain. My mind cried out, demanding to know where this all-knowing, intervening God was when my father was ending his life. Why hadn't God sent an angel to cry out to stop him, as God did when Abraham was about to sacrifice Isaac (Genesis 22:11–12)? I listened to the prayer *Ufros aleinu sukkat sh'lomecha*—"Spread over us Your shelter of shalom."[2] In my anger I wanted to know—why hadn't God done that for my father? Standing inside the sanctuary, I found no comfort. The liturgy only fueled my anger and my questions. The only prayers that I could offer came in the form of my tears.[3] It was simply too hard to be there. So I stopped going. And as I stepped away, the space between me, God, and my faith grew wider. How terribly lonely it felt to lose God, just when I needed Them most.[4] It compounded my grief. In Psalm 23:4, we read, "Though I walk through a valley of the shadow of death, I will fear no evil, for You are with me." But I was afraid, and I felt alone. This valley, this foreign and difficult terrain, so new and endless, overwhelmed me, and the only things that connected me to the God of my faith were my yells, my silence, and my cries.

Rabbi David Wolpe shared recently in a blog post, "We are spatially oriented creatures. Although love, justice, mathematics, and other accompaniments of life exist apart from physicality, God remains difficult to separate in our thoughts from notions of place."[5] This is where I found myself for many years after my father's death. Slowly and continually wandering the valley of the shadows, navigating the difficult terrain of traumatic grief, I found no spiritual grounding when my knees began to buckle. If I could not return to synagogue, to that notion of place where I had been taught that God dwelled, how could I be in relationship with the Divine? Where could I find the words that reflected what was in my heart?

> Oh God, I search for you.
> Amidst the fragments, the shattered pieces, the mess that's
>   left behind.
> This journey through the valley of the shadows feels so dark,
>   so long, so unfamiliar.
> I wonder.
> Are you with me, God?

I search and I yearn, but I do not feel you.
I long to be enveloped in your loving arms.
I long to know that my father is in your care.
I long to know that he is at peace.
I long to know that one day I will be too.
Adonai, be my compass.
Help me to reach toward life, toward hope, toward renewal.
Help me to begin again.
Hear my cries.
Comfort me, oh God.
Comfort me as a parent, for I am a child in pain.
Help me to see you, to feel you, to know your presence.[6]

These words are my own. They are a part of a prayer that I wrote on November 19, 2015, seven months after my father's death. I had always found writing to be a great salve, a way to breathe life into what I was feeling. Writing about suicide loss and grief became a vehicle of healing for me, and as I published my reflections on my blog, they soon found their way to other sites and forums. My words connected me to others who had lost a loved one to suicide. They would write to me and share their experiences. Many offered gratitude that I was not allowing shame or stigma to keep me from sharing my experience. I was cultivating a community that allowed me to feel seen and understood, but more than that, I was creating a place where I could give voice to the prayers of my heart. If the liturgy of my faith didn't speak to my pain or bring me comfort, I decided that I would create and share my own.

The journey through grief
So vast, dark and uncertain
Where is my compass
God, are you with me
I search, eyes closed, heart open
Oh Source of comfort
I cry out in tears
A primal ache in my soul
Help me to find you[7]

These were the conversations I began to have with God as I traversed the valley, doing the hard work of grieving out loud. Slowly, I realized that there was an intimacy expressed in these words. At the time, I am not sure that I felt I was in conversation with God. But I began to allow for the notion that my words, still separate from the sacred place of the synagogue, might be reaching Something larger than myself. And just as importantly, I was helping to cultivate a new language of solace— prayers and reflections around traumatic grief and suicide loss—that hadn't been available to me. That, too, expanded my notion of what it means to be a part of Jewish communal spaces, even if the most obvious one felt too hard to enter.

As I sit here today, I can see with great clarity how far I have traveled through this wilderness of traumatic loss. I've been on this journey for many years now. When I began, the weight of all that I carried left me barely able to stand. But slowly, and sometimes without even noticing, the load began to lighten. Somewhere along the way, I was able to let go of the guilt and the unanswerable question of why. Further along the path, I learned to forgive my father and relinquish my anger at him. I unpacked all the signs until I knew his "emotional autopsy" by heart. Only after that was I able to forgive myself for being unable to see all that my father hid from me. And as I stood at my father's grave, just before COVID-19 brought the world to a halt, I even forgave God—though until now, I don't think I understood what that meant.

In my mind, even in forgiveness, I still held a certain image of my relationship with God. I pictured the two of us sitting across a great chasm from one another, neither of us speaking, neither of us attempting to bridge that divide, and both of us left without a language to communicate. Traditional liturgy and prayer still felt too painful for me. If I dared to speak to an intervening or almighty God, I'd never be able to forgive Them for not intervening to help my father. In the earliest years of my grief, I knew the language of railing at God, hurling all my pain and anger at Them, wailing in tears, placing all of my suffering on Their shoulders—not necessarily because They were deserving of it, but because I needed someplace to put it. But after I forgave God, that no longer seemed a tenable or meaningful mode of communication. So, what was I left with?

This standoff image of God and me across the chasm remained in my mind. I was unable to rely on texts and song or the raw, spewing language of grief. How were we to be engaged in this relationship? We just sat. It appeared stagnant. Maybe irrevocably broken. Neither of us said anything, yet neither of us moved away or turned our backs. That same question came to mind again, the one I had asked my husband sitting at our bedside in those first days of grief: "Would it ever feel better than it did at that moment? Would I ever learn to have faith and trust in God, as my loving and constant companion? Or would I only know God as a figment, unreachable, unknowable to me, always just too far out of my reach?"

It is only now that I have finally come to see that my relationship with God and my faith was never about the liturgy or the songs. Those are things that tie me to my people, to my heritage, but I do not find comfort in them anymore because they do not reflect the God that sits across from me. If they did, God would've constructed a bridge across the chasm. God would've carried me across the valley of shadows and given me confirmation that I wasn't alone. God would've sent me a sign that my father was okay and at peace. God would've woken me with a crash of thunder and a deep sense of foreboding that might've allowed me to intervene in my father's plans for death. But that is not the God that sits across from me. That is not the God I ever believed in, even when the liturgy said differently.

Sitting across this great chasm, facing one another, and not speaking a word—this is exactly what it means to be in a relationship with one another.

In that same blog post, Rabbi Wolpe shares, "The building of the mishkan did not change God, but it changed Israel. It taught us to both seek out and create spaces where we can feel God's presence. God may be the same everywhere, but we are not."[8]

This is the very essence of faith. God has stayed with me, patiently waiting, facing me with a willingness to hold whatever I hurled across the way. God has never once turned and walked away or offered me Their back, and neither have I. We have stayed engaged simply by continually occupying that space. This whole time, God and I have stayed in a relationship with one another. My prayers came in soft utterances and guttural cries. They came in angry torrents, cuss words, and silent treatments. And God listened to them all, while we remained across the divide. But the point is that we both remained. God had not changed. But I had.

I know now that the chasm is not insurmountable or in need of an object, a moment, a shift in the universe to bring us together. The chasm is the seeking. It is the space into which you can hurl the ideas and ideals that get in the way. I tossed into it the notion that God could've saved my father with an outstretched hand. Now I choose to believe that God was with him in his final moments to ease his suffering and tend to his wounds. I have learned that you can stand at the edge and surrender to the unknowable and uncontrollable and open yourself instead to the belief that whatever comes, you won't go through it alone. God will surround you with love. Into the abyss, let go of the childhood stories of the God that rescued, and therefore must've also abandoned, Their children. Instead, search for God in the tiny miracles and moments of grace. The chasm, the space between, isn't a fault line or a sinkhole. The chasm doesn't mean that my faith is broken. The chasm is the journey, whether we leap across it or expand our reach, whether we circle around it or simply sit with it. So long as we keep showing up, we are with God. God never left me, nor did They leave my father.

My faith is not broken. This journey has not broken me. I carry my wounds in this relationship, just as I do with others. They are a part of my story, a personal liturgy. I find God in the open spaces and the quiet moments. I find God in the whisper of the wind and the cries I still offer for my father. God and I remain engaged across the chasm. I am learning to trust that no matter the journey, I can cleave to the belief that we will not abandon one another. We never have. It's taken me a while to figure that out. But perhaps that too is part of the process of healing.

I have not made peace with the prayers or even with most of the liturgy. But, throughout this journey, I have been a seeker. Sometimes it can be one sentence, a singular image, or a new perspective that allows me to connect my experience with the words and teachings of our sacred sources. Those instances allow me to engage with these words differently and openly. Psalm 121:1–2 says, "I lift my eyes to the mountains; from where will my help come? My help will come from God." Another name for God is *HaMakom*, "the place." I can let that divine presence in, no matter where my feet stand. The place, the holiest sanctuary, lies within. It is not composed of four walls or even an ark. And when I need to look outward to be reminded of a healing presence, I can look to the beautiful Colorado mountains in this place that I call home. That too is a place of divine encounter. God was with me in the valley and has accompanied me through the trails, the peaks, and the plateaus. And this place, this chasm that we call home, is holy ground.

NOTES

1. The *Kaddish*, also known as *Kaddish Yatom* or the Mourner's Kaddish, is a prayer focused on God's greatness and goodness and is recited daily for a year after a loss and on the anniversary of a loss.

2. *Hashkiveinu*, *Mishkan T'filah: For Weekdays, Shabbat, Festivals and other occasions of public worship* (CCAR Press, 2007), 160. Babylonian Talmud, *Bava M'tzia* 59a, "Although the gates of prayer are locked, the gates of tears are not."

4. I choose to use "They/Them/Theirs" as God's pronouns, reflecting God's nonbinary nature.

5. David Wolpe, "Terumah—The Space Inside Us," *Impressions: A Rabbi's Commentary and Contemplation* (blog), February 15, 2024. https://www.sinaitemple.org/learn/rabbi-wolpe-adl-impressions/terumah-the-space-inside-of-us/.

6. Deborah L. Greene, "A Survivor's Prayer," *Reflecting Out Loud* (blog), November 19, 2015, https://reflectingoutloud.net/2015/11/19/a-survivors-prayer/.

7. Deborah L. Greene, "Grief in Haiku," *Reflecting Out Loud* (blog), January 22, 2016, https://reflectingoutloud.net/2016/01/22/grief-in-haiku/.

8. Wolpe, "Terumah."

38

The Crawl Space Between Grief and Gratitude

The Devastating Death of a Daughter

Rabbi Susan Talve

Maybe that's what the crawl space is between grief and gratitude—remembrance or memory.
—*Adina Talve-Goodman,* Your Hearts, Your Scars

WHEN NAOMI RETURNED home with Ruth by her side, she was welcomed by name. She replied, "Do not call me Naomi [pleas-ant one]. Call me Mara [bitter], for Shaddai has made my lot very bitter. I went away full and the Eternal has brought me back empty" (Ruth 1:20–21).[1] The Biblical Book of Ruth tells of love and loyalty in the face of profound loss. Naomi and her family leave their home to escape famine and go to the land of the hated Moabites. There, her sons marry Moabite women, Ruth and Orpah. When Naomi's husband and sons die, she decides to return home, and she encourages her daughters-in-law to return to their families. However, Ruth is determined to stay with Naomi, her beloved mother-in-law. Ruth's selfless act of devotion leads to redemption for the family and the Jewish people through the birth of her child with her second husband, Boaz. Ruth's descendants belong to the Davidic messianic line.

The deaths of her husband and two sons left Naomi in a state of grief: bitter and empty. I used to believe that Ruth was Naomi's healing, that Ruth's love and loyalty could fill that empty space as well as secure the future. Now I know better. The death of my child has left me bitter and empty. The harsh edges may soften over time, and the steady flow of tears may dry, but the space she left is filled with the trauma of her death and the pain of grief.

Adina, our third child in four years, was born on December 12, 1986. We rejoiced with humility and gratitude at the birth of another healthy child. My husband and I are both rabbis, and we had witnessed all that could go wrong; I learned to expect the worst. During my pregnancy, I stood with our foremother Rebekah and cried out to the universe, "*Im kein, lamah zeh anochi?*" (If this, why am I?) (Genesis 25:22).[2] Like Rebekah, I was scared. Through my lens of fear I interpreted her question as, "If this is reality, where life is fragile and there is the awful possibility of a mother or child dying, and the world is broken and fraught with the many dangers we expose our vulnerable children to, what is the point?" And then, for a moment, the world was working as it should. I remember the doctor saying, "After all that worry, another healthy child."

At nine hours old, our pediatrician noticed a blueness around our perfect child's mouth. "We need to take a closer look," she told us. At twelve hours old, Adina received her first invasive procedure. By twenty-four hours old, she had had her first of many heart surgeries, her first of many scars. And from her first breath we were madly in love, our souls bound with hers.

We gave her the name Adina because she was so *adin*, so delicate and beautiful. We added the name Chaya, for a great-grandmother's protection and for a long life. We sensed we were entering a world that would change us and demand a deep spiritual practice to respond in holy ways to the challenges that would unfold.

The congregation I helped found was only two years old when Adina was born, but helping my family became their mission. I didn't have maternity leave with our first two children, born in the early 1980s, but this new congregation would create a different model. We were going to be feminist and egalitarian and open and affirming. When Adina was well enough and I was finally able to come back to work, the congregation asked what more they could do. I remember answering, "If we could do for each other what you have done for my family and me, we will grow the beloved community we are reaching for." The Central Reform Congregation Mitzvah Corps, a sophisticated service initiative within the congregation that has saved and changed lives, was born alongside Adina. Forty years later, it continues to be part of her legacy.

Despite her many surgeries and scars, Adina had a charmed life. She delighted everyone with her beauty, her brilliance, and her humor. She excelled at everything she touched. She won a prestigious writing prize for her essay "I Must Have Been That Man" in 2017. This profound piece uses a well-known Talmudic story that asks the question, "Are your sufferings dear to you?" (Babylonian Talmud, *B'rachot* 5b). The answer in the story: "Not they nor their reward."

Her father and I were always surprised and delighted when she referenced stories and images from Jewish tradition. We told her this one just before her heart transplant in 2006. After running a support group for families and children born with congenital heart disease for twenty years, I knew that "heart kids" often became attached to illnesses that make their accomplishments heroic. Many posttransplant recipients who live with "normal hearts" for the first time cannot handle being well. They are used to being heroes living with suffering and many challenges to overcome. We wanted Adina to know that she was a gifted and remarkable human being in spite of, not because of, the challenges brought about by her illness.

The story won her a place at the University of Iowa's renowned Master of Fine Arts (MFA) program for nonfiction to work on more pieces about living with bodies of difference and trauma. After her first year in the program, Adina was diagnosed with a rare form of cancer caused by the immunosuppressant drugs she was taking to prevent the rejection of her new heart. She came home to receive treatments that we were told would "cure" her cancer. We believed that this was just another bump in the road because she had survived worse. I had faith that she would defy the angel of death again.

I am an activist rabbi. The practice of responding to the suffering around me is deeply rooted in the liturgy and teachings that inform my understanding of Judaism. Building relationships with others who share these values and fighting together to overcome the disparities in health care, housing, education, and economic mobility deepen my faith daily. I started a statewide health-care coalition and was a regular member of the "protest family," marching and working for racial justice. I was drawn into the streets with this family even before Adina was born, by the cries of mothers losing their children to police and gun violence. When Adina was diagnosed with cancer, we were protesting another unjust verdict of a police officer who was not being held accountable for the death of another young Black man.

As the protests unfolded and we entered the awful world of cancer with our daughter, I had to step back from fighting racism and injustice and take my place fighting the broken "sick care" system for the life of my child. Adina did everything asked of her so that she could return to the life she loved with her family and her friends. She did not like the violent "war" language used by so many when discussing cancer. It was not about fighting, winning, or losing for Adina. She just wanted to be strong and healthy again. Activism is often led by those who hope for the opportunity to live lives of equity and to be treated fairly—no more, no less.

On January 12, 2018, just as Shabbat was beginning, Adina died unexpectedly from an infection. With her last breath, she looked at me and whispered, "I love you." I went into shock, but I knew what to do from the countless times I had been with families at the moment their loved ones died. I comforted my children, called the funeral home, and texted family who would need to come quickly. I made decisions about organ donation. My husband and I sent everyone home.

I crawled into bed with her and held her body until the transport people came. We accompanied the body through the bowels of the hospital until they put her in their SUV and drove off. I made sure that there would be a *shomeir*,[3] a "guard," with the body at all times. I live in the trauma of that awful moment every day, always wondering what more I could have done, what stone we had left unturned. The last hours of her life play and replay in my mind. I don't remember if I also said, "I love you."

Living with pain requires daily spiritual practice. Staying connected to the cycles of the moon, the study of the weekly Torah portion, and intentionally practicing Jewish principles—such as loving-kindness, giving the benefit of the doubt, generosity, and deep listening—continue to pick me up from my pain and push me forward.

Sh'mot, the Torah portion that we were reading the week Adina died, describes how God is drawn into the story of Pesach by the groans of the enslaved Israelites. The week of her funeral and shivah took us through the plagues and the awful price of freedom inflicted on the Egyptians, who also lost their children. I remember thinking that Adina was teaching me humility. As lonely as grief is, my tradition and my practice remind me that I am not alone. There are others who understand the unthinkable loss of a child and will not try to fix my guilt and my grief. The week of the first cycle of the moon without Adina was *T'rumah*, the portion that describes how God tells the people to "make Me a sanctuary" (Exodus 25:8) so that we may never again be trapped by the illusion that we are separate from God. The teachings of each Torah portion dragged me through that first year and continue to guide me to this day.

When the first High Holy Days came, I was back on the bimah, still tender and teary. I spoke about the idiom "at the mercy of," a phrase that describes being vulnerable and defenseless. In the Jewish tradition, to be "at the mercy of" something is to be without a protective cover. This is because the Torah teaches in the Book of Exodus that a *kaporet*, translated as "seat of mercy," rests above the Ark. The Torah describes a lid made of pure gold and decorated with two cherubim that formed the cover to the Ark that held the teachings of God. This artistic cover formed a space or seat upon which God's presence could dwell—hence, the "seat of mercy" (Exodus 25:17–22). This seat of mercy allows us to be vulnerable and still safe because the cover protects us.

The root of *kaporet*, the cover that keeps us safe, comes from the same Hebrew root—*kaf-pei-reish*—that forms the second word in "Yom Kippur" and the word for atonement (*kaparah*). If we repent on this day, if we truly change our ways, then godliness and goodness and glory will fill the seat of mercy, and the two cherubim that surround the seat—one that stands for justice and the other for mercy—will integrate and put the world in a better balance so that we will be less vulnerable and less "at the mercy of" brokenness and suffering.

What is this mercy we need to fill that seat with? In Hebrew mercy is *rachamim*, from *rechem*, the word for womb—something so primal, so vulnerable, so deep inside. In English, the word "mercy" is from the Latin *misericordia*. *Miserere* is "to pity," and *cor* is "heart." Together, they suggest that mercy means to have a heart for someone's troubles; to have mercy is to care.

In her book *Hallelujah Anyway: Rediscovering Mercy*, Anne Lamott suggests that mercy is not something you do, but instead is something within that needs to be cultivated, like a muscle.[4] This aligns with the Hebrew word for mercy, *rachamim*. Whether you have a literal womb or not, to have mercy is to feel the pain of others enough to have to try to do something about it. To cultivate mercy is to take the time to really listen, to care enough to learn about others, and to be part of the cover that protects the most vulnerable. Practicing this as an act of radical kindness helps me to honor my daughter's memory and help to make it a blessing.

There are times when we are also at the mercy of our own individual limitations. I may want to do more, but I am at the mercy of my energy, my limited wisdom, and my grief. I am often paralyzed by the mistakes I have made, the opportunities I have missed, and the people I have let down. This makes me afraid to try again. It makes me doubt that I can trust myself and others again. Sometimes—oftentimes—the circumstances of our lives that are beyond our control really do have us at their mercy. Anyone who has cared for a loved one who has died knows what it is to live at the mercy of these limitations.

One of the things I most appreciate about Jewish tradition is that our heroes are far from perfect. Our heroes are also at the mercy of their limitations. Abraham's selective justice leads him to come close to killing both of his sons and sets up generations of dysfunction and trauma, while also arguing that an entire city be saved for the sake of ten innocent people. Sarah's jealousy causes the cruel casting out of Hagar and her son Ishmael into the wilderness, while also welcoming so many into her tent. Rebekah and Jacob play favorites with their children, pitting them against each other, continuing the generational trauma they had each suffered. Moses, Miriam, David, and my spirit-sister Naomi are all portrayed with character flaws—each of them, like so many of us, is far from perfect.

Each of our heroes gives us lessons on being at the mercy of our limitations. They teach us to avoid making the same mistakes and accept that we, too, are flawed. They help us live with our limitations and encourage us to try and be better. They dare us to be humble enough to keep trying in the face of all we have endured, all we have been at the mercy of. Despite everything, we keep believing that we can fill that heavenly seat through our atonement and that mercy will overflow. We have faith that we can keep trying to make things better for all of us.

A few months after Adina died, when I could barely leave our house,

I went to the US–Mexico border. I heard the cries of the children separated from their parents, and I had to respond. It felt so personal.

I felt the fear of parents who had already made dangerous journeys to save their lives and the lives of their children and were now at the mercy of a system that has no empathy for their families. I went to put my body on the line in a protest against the policies of Immigration and Customs Enforcement (ICE) in San Diego. Everyone impacted was at the mercy of systems that were so out of balance they were causing trauma for the workers as well as for the immigrants, refugees, and their children. We learned that children, no matter how much kindness they are shown, will never forget and most likely never forgive being torn from their parents' arms. Memory also fills the crawl space with trauma.

There are also many beautiful memories that have crept into the crawl space Adina dared us to inhabit between grief and gratitude. There are moments we who are bruised and broken share with a smile.

I often think about the Talmudic story I mentioned above that asks, "Are your sufferings dear to you?" and answers, "Not they nor their reward." In Adina's story, she answers, "Maybe just a little." At first, I wasn't sure what she meant, but I continue to learn from my daughter. Yes, my sufferings are dear to me too. The pain of losing her and my grief keep Adina close.

Living with my failings and limitations continues to be humbling in a chaotic and disappointing world. The teachings of Torah, the holidays, and the spiritual practice demanded by prayer and Shabbat drag me forward into each new day trying to be a better person. I am continually surprised by a faith that keeps me trying to bring more mercy into the world and honoring the gift of being Adina's mother, until—I can only hope—I will be with her again.

NOTES

1. *The JPS Tanakh: Gender-Sensitive Edition* (Jewish Publication Society, 2023), found on Sefaria (sefaria.org).

2. In Genesis 25:22–24 we learn that Rebekah is pregnant with twins, who are struggling in her womb. I imagine how frightened and worried she must have been for her life and the lives of her babies as she faces childbirth. This remarkable moment is preserved as this brave woman calls

out to God, asking for the purpose of her life in the face of such uncertainty. God's response is also preserved. Translated by the author.

3. It is a Jewish tradition to make sure that the body is never alone between death and the burial. A *shomeir* (guard) is employed to sit with the body, out of respect.

4. Anne Lammot, *Hallelujah Anyway: Rediscovering Mercy* (Penguin, 2017).

39

A Path to Healing Through Tradition

Jewish Mourning Rituals and Beliefs After the Death of My Child

Rabbi Rex D. Perlmeter, LSW

"Hi, I'm Rex. My son died." Perhaps it wasn't quite that austere, but for a long while, that was the essence of almost every conversation in which I engaged. The volume of detail (and tears) was usually dependent upon the nature and level of the relationship, be it family, friends, colleagues, or acquaintances (new or old). In the end, there was one message: "My son died." This was the case from the day of Mitch's death—February 1, 2011—for a good couple of years. During that time, our loss was absolutely the central narrative of my life.[1] After came a period of a few years of pulsing between that narrative and other, happier threads that were taking shape in my life. Finally, in the last few years, I have found myself living primarily in a space of joy and abundance in my personal, professional, and avocational lives. The cloud of grief, but also the radiant outline of that cloud that is the living presence of Mitch's love, are always present—usually in the background, but sometimes center stage again for a time. I offer this chronicle of my journey and the crucial role, themes, and rubrics of Jewish mourning tradition in the prayer that it will bless others traveling their own journeys, with the hope that such possibility exists for them as well.

Aninut

Our world came crashing to a halt on that morning in 2011 when Mitch collapsed in the shower as the result of an undiagnosed cardiac condition. The moment he was pronounced dead in the emergency room, we entered the period our tradition calls *aninut*. When I speak with families immediately after a death, I translate this as "bereavement," distinct from "mourning." In Jewish teaching, bereavement encompasses the period from death to burial. It is a period during which one is exempt from observing the mitzvot (actions required by Jewish law) and during which those outside the immediate circle of loss are not supposed to visit or even try to comfort the bereaved. I've always thought this showed that the shapers of our tradition had a profound understanding of the nature of shock—a state that Emily Dickinson describes so accurately in this poem:

> After great pain, a formal feeling comes—
> The Nerves sit ceremonious, like Tombs—
> The stiff Heart questions 'was it He, that bore,'
> And 'Yesterday, or Centuries before'?
>
> The Feet, mechanical, go round—
> A Wooden way
> Of Ground, or Air, or Ought—
> Regardless grown,
> A Quartz contentment, like a stone—
>
> This is the Hour of Lead—
> Remembered, if outlived,
> As Freezing persons, recollect the Snow—
> First—Chill—then Stupor—then the letting go—[2]

If you've been there, you'll know the place Dickinson is describing, and you may have experienced that stupor. In the first hours and days following Mitch's death, I was so raw, I could barely tolerate any contact or action that required acknowledging that I was even alive. The grace of the *aninut* period was a gift of acknowledgment that my world had ground to a halt.

There is one moment during this period that stands out amid the all-encompassing darkness and fog. The morning after Mitch's death, I found myself wishing away the length of days I could reasonably expect to have as a white, affluent man living in twenty-first-century America (with a full understanding of the privilege of that expectation). Having always been excited by the idea of perhaps living into triple digits (to 120?!), I suddenly experienced dread at the thought of decades without Mitch's enveloping hugs. It must have shown on my face, because when I came out of the bathroom, my wife, Rachel, took one look at me and said, "We can't live in the world of what might have been; we have to live in the world of what is." This mindfulness-informed teaching from someone who had not yet studied mindfulness practice became pivotal for me. It guided me to a new commitment to the oft-quoted mandate from the Torah *Uvacharta bachayim*, "Choose life" (Deuteronomy 30:19). In that moment, I understood that a choice was available to me, and I made the choice to somehow go on living, with the hope that one day it could and would again be with fullness of heart. In noting this, I want to acknowledge the blessing of temperament. I know myself to be hardwired for joy and positive, sometimes even impulsive, energy. Choosing life was made easier by that hardwiring, and we should never fall into the trap of judging those for whom that choice is more difficult. Rather, it is our task to help build a world that feels worth choosing.

L'vayat HaMeit and Shivah

Mitch's funeral and burial remain somewhat of a blur. By the time of the service, I was ready to tear the ribbon of mourning and utter the fatal words *Baruch Dayan ha-emet* (Blessed be the righteous Judge). I was too angry to do so when our friend and rabbi, Steven Kushner, arrived at the hospital just as we were leaving Mitch's side. To me, in that moment, the words promised that one day I would make meaning out of this senseless tragedy, but that felt a long way off. That meaning began to glimmer in the beautiful and spot-on eulogy Steve offered and in the outpouring of love and supportive strength offered by the hundreds of people with us that day. Because we knew we would not be able to handle a prolonged time in the cemetery waiting to bury him, we did that privately, surrounded by our very closest friends and family who had been and would continue to be our immediate lifeline. While all else is indistinct, one memory remains clear—that of our dear friend Joanie Berger starting a circle of loved ones holding hands and singing *Oseh Shalom* (Maker of Peace) around Mitch's final resting place. This was truly a *l'vayat hameit*, an accompaniment of Mitch's beautiful body to its final home, even as we began to release our hold on his *n'shamah*, his soul, to return to its ultimate Home.

Shivah, the seven-day period of intense mourning—in our case a multiday open house for receiving visits of consolation and worshiping in our home rather than in the synagogue—is also hazy in memory. It was, frankly, exhausting—but also warm, loving, and often funny.

Mitch's friends had many great anecdotes to share, which delighted and sometimes surprised us. The love was obviously vital and healing, and I learned that the exhaustion was as well. The latter maintained the helpful numbing that cushions us as we move into the deepest wells of grief. This pairing of tradition and psychology seems to me, again, brilliant and benevolent. By the time shivah was over, we were ready for it to be over (especially our kids!), and reluctantly, we were preparing ourselves to begin the task of survival and, possibly, healing.

The *Kaddish* Year and My *Shiviti*

With the end of shivah, we moved into both the first year of mourning and our status as mourners, called upon to recite *Kaddish Yatom*, the Mourner's *Kaddish* (the prayer of praise to the Holy One that is recited in memory of our dead). The practice of *Kaddish* was important for me on multiple levels, and I began to think of the practice in new ways. First, the opportunity to recite the prayer in community was critical. Feeling ourselves held by our congregational family provided a cocoon in which we could begin to regrow our wings. Our temple, like many, had already adopted the practice of inviting mourners to share the names of their beloveds. Naming Mitch and being recognized in my grief was deeply meaningful; I felt seen in my suffering, and I needed that. I am happy to see more of our congregations altering the early Reform practice of everyone standing and all reciting this *Kaddish* together. Most congregations in which I've worshiped in recent years now invite mourners to stand first and then invite the congregation to rise in support. It feels right and needed. Mourning is a unique category of being and deserves to be known as such. In the years since Mitch's death, I have adopted the more traditional practice of reciting only the communal responses in the recitation and leaving the mourners the space to recite the full text, with support as and when needed. As a family of two Reform rabbis and their children, all with lifelong involvement in the Reform Movement and its institutions (e.g., synagogues and camps), we had the blessing of that support not only from our congregation but from a worldwide network. During the first month, we knew that Mitch's name was being recited around the globe. What a gift, through our affiliation, to be part of so large and loving a world!

Kaddish was also important as a way to remain mindful of the special status and limits that come with the mourning period. Our tradition clearly limits the period for mourners to recite *Kaddish*. In the case of a child, the limit is a month, which I completely disregarded. I needed the year to fully move out of the space of mourning and into the space of living. By limiting the time we can recite *Kaddish*, our tradition conveys that message. It does not deny the permanence of grief but invites us to move from living *in* grief to living *with* grief. The limits are arbitrary, and indeed my phase of acute mourning lasted longer than a year, but having a limit taught me to recognize that at some point I would need and would be able to make that move. And we are invited by our practice to ritually renew our acquaintance with the grief for the losses we carry five times a year—on the four occasions of communal *Yizkor* (remembrance), as well as on the *yahrzeit* (the anniversary of the death). Grief is invited to have a place, but not to remain our whole world. Once again, *uvacharta bachayim*—"choose life."

Kaddish also helped me structure my days in that first year. My practice was not in accordance with halachah (Jewish law), in that I did not attend daily minyan.[3] At the time, I was commuting from New Jersey to New York City. It was hard enough for me to get up in time to catch my train (okay, I often ended up catching the one after my train). But I did get into the habit of reciting *Kaddish* quietly every morning on the train and took great comfort from this practice. One piece of the practice was especially meaningful to me. There is a Jewish mystical object called a *shiviti*. It is a piece of word art centered around a verse from Psalm 16:8, which says, *Shiviti Adonai l'negdi tamid*, "I have set the Eternal always before me." The *shiviti* is used as an object of contemplation to help us see that there is truly no place or entity in this Creation where God is absent. Every morning, before reciting *Kaddish*, I would open my iPad to my home-screen photo—a picture of Mitch, about three months before his death, sitting on a beach with his huge toothy smile. A lifeguard tower looms behind him, suggesting to me that Mitch, in the embrace of the Eternal, is watching over all of us. This *shiviti* continues to give me great comfort to this day. And during those early days, this was my window into God, as pointed out to me by my treasured colleague and spiritual director Myriam Klotz. I was still too raw and angry to approach God directly in those months, but through Mitch, I could feel the river of *chesed* (loving-kindness) in which the Holy One manifests in this world, and I could feel held. May all who mourn know that feeling.

T'chiyat HaMeitim

This brings me to another theme embodied in a practice, *t'chiyat hameitim* (revival of the dead). During that first year, I changed my recitation of the second blessing in the *Amidah* (the central set of blessings in Jewish worship). As practiced in the Reform Judaism of my first five decades, we would recite, *Baruch atah Adonai . . . m'chayeih hakol*, "Blessed are You, Adonai . . . who gives life to all." Within a few weeks of Mitch's death, I began reciting the more traditional version of the blessing, *m'chayeih hameitim*, "who revives the dead." That statement of faith held true for me as I began to feel myself returning to life and to a semblance of who I was before his death. The textual change was meaningful to me in another sense as well. Mitch was palpably present to me for much of those first couple of years after his death. I had a general feeling of his spirit hovering near and at times particularly strong—even physical—sensations of a presence, which I knew to be his. As I often said in speaking engagements, it is fully conceivable to me that this might have been a grief psychosis, and I don't care. Regardless of the source, it gave me much needed comfort and joy. In the years since, that presence has largely receded. I believe a part of Mitch remained close for the time when it was most needed here, and now he dwells fully in the Oneness of which we are all a part, though still making the occasional visit. We are the stuff of eternity.

There even came a point at which that presence, as it were, spoke to me. Like many survivors of traumatic loss, I carried a burden of guilt. I was in the room directly beneath the bathroom where Mitch breathed his last. In my innermost depths, I would berate myself: How could I have sat calmly reading my newspaper and drinking my coffee while my son was dying? How could I have missed the signs and failed to save him? And one morning, about two years after he died, I felt him come to me, and the words arose within me, "Dad," in that slightly exasperated way he would sometimes say it, "it's okay. It's all peace." Nothing more, but that was a release that healed a major tear in my soul, and I believed and still believe it with my whole heart. As our liturgy says, *B'yado afkid ruchi b'eit ishan v'a-irah, v'im ruchi g'viyati; Adonai li, v'lo ira*, "I place my spirit in Your hand and my physical being as well, when I lie down and when I rise up; the Eternal is with me, I will not fear."

Uvacharta BaChayim

That is where and how I now dwell, at least most of the time. In the words of Rami Shapiro, I know myself to be "loved by an Unending Love,"[4] and Mitch is deeply part of that Love. There are still moments of deep sadness, but my surviving family is thriving and living life to the fullest. Mitch's death is now part of our narrative, but it is not the whole. A few months after his death, Rachel and I acquired a painting titled *Misty Sun*, depicting a multihued, hazy sky through which the light of the star at the heart of our solar system penetrates and lends warmth. Instead of a black hole at the center of our family's universe, Mitch's presence and memory are now a light that radiates through the fog of loss and memory to bring warmth and gratitude to every day of our lives. *Zichrono livrachah*—his memory is the greatest of blessings.

Notes

1. I write throughout this chapter in the first-person singular, as I do not presume to speak on behalf of my wife and colleague, Rachel Hertzman, or our surviving children, Jackie, Sarah, and Nate. Each of us had our own deep pit of personal devastation in the wake of Mitch's death, and each traveled their own, mutually supportive journey out of the pit of despair. I honor their journeys and the love with which we have accompanied one another.

2. Emily Dickinson, "After great pain a formal feeling comes" from *The Poems of Emily Dickinson: Reading Edition*, edited by Ralph W. Franklin, Cambridge, Mass.: The Belknap Press of Harvard University Press, Copyright © 1998, 1999 by the President and Fellows of Harvard College. Copyright © 1951, 1955 by the President and Fellows of Harvard College. Copyright © renewed 1979, 1983 by the President and Fellows of Harvard College. Copyright © 1914, 1918, 1919, 1924, 1929, 1930, 1932, 1935, 1937, 1942 by Martha Dickinson Bianchi. Copyright © 1952, 1957, 1958, 1963, 1965 by Mary L. Hampson. Used by permission. All rights reserved.

3. A minyan is a group of ten Jews; ten is the minimum number of people required to be in attendance at a worship service in order to recite certain prayers including the Mourner's Kaddish.
4. Rami Shapiro, "Unending Love," in *Beside Still Waters: A Journey of Comfort and Renewal*, ed. Rachel Barenblat (Ben Yehuda Press, 2019), 74.

Nechemta: Finding Comfort

RABBI LINDSEY DANZIGER

Okay, DEEP BREATH. Inhale. Exhale.

Thank you for engaging with the stories of trauma, resilience, and ultimately of hope shared by the authors in the previous pages. By bearing witness to the experiences of others and, hopefully, by learning alongside us and our journeys, you have walked in sacred presence and acknowledgment of some of the darkest moments in our lives. That knowledge brings me healing, fights against the toxic loneliness of trauma, and hopefully will touch many of this volume's authors in a similar way.

It is also important to take care of yourself after wading through the heavy content of this book. Secondary trauma is the emotional distress caused by bearing witness to the trauma of others, and we urge you to take notice of how your body and emotions react to the stories on these pages. This book is written so that you are able to step away for as long as you need and then come back to this volume when it serves you in a way that cares for your own well-being.

Along with our trauma, deep in the Jewish psyche and ingrained into the Jewish experience is the muscle of hope. We have flexed and conditioned it over generations. It has been necessary to utilize anew in both surprising and unsurprising ways in each of our lives. The old joke goes: What is the difference between the Jewish pessimist and the Jewish optimist? The pessimists says, "It can't possibly get any worse." And the optimist replies, "Sure it can!" Our history is an anthology not just of the traumas our textual ancestors and our people have shared and experienced individually, but of their creative and enlightening responses to these challenges. Person by person, community by community, we have added our own stories of trial and resilience to the archaeology of struggle that came before, learning from them and adding our own teachings for those who come after. We hope these pages have been an addition to the collective wisdom that guides our hearts and our minds. Our heritage and collective memory remind us that while we journey through experiences that threaten to break us, we are not alone. We are joined by those who came before us, sharing their wisdom in our sacred texts, in our history, and in the bravery of sharing our own stories.

We began the early conversations about this book right as the COVID-19 pandemic was emerging, and I am penning this final chapter in September 2024, one week after the bodies of six Israeli hostages, including American Israeli Hersh Goldberg-Polin, were found executed in a tunnel below Gaza just one day after they had been alive. The trauma of this moment frankly feels paralyzing. Hersh, and his mother in particular, have served as beacons of hope during this bleak time of despair and cycle of destruction. Rachel Goldberg-Polin has emerged as a matriarch and teacher of the Jewish people, processing her trauma publicly and serving as an example and lesson in resilience for us all. With the murder of her son, so close to the possibility of his rescue, we all crashed into the trauma that comes with sudden loss of hope.

Thus said God:	כֹּה אָמַר יְיָ
A cry is heard in Ramah—	קוֹל בְּרָמָה נִשְׁמָע
Wailing, bitter weeping—	נְהִי בְּכִי תַמְרוּרִים
Rachel weeping for her children.	רָחֵל מְבַכָּה עַל־בָּנֶיהָ
She refuses to be comforted	מֵאֲנָה לְהִנָּחֵם
For her children, who are gone.	עַל־בָּנֶיהָ כִּי אֵינֶנּוּ:
Thus said God:	כֹּה אָמַר יְיָ
Restrain your voice from weeping,	מִנְעִי קוֹלֵךְ מִבֶּכִי
Your eyes from shedding tears;	וְעֵינַיִךְ מִדִּמְעָה
For there is a reward for your labor	כִּי יֵשׁ שָׂכָר לִפְעֻלָּתֵךְ
—declares God:	נְאֻם־יְיָ
They shall return from the enemy's land.	וְשָׁבוּ מֵאֶרֶץ אוֹיֵב:
And there is hope for your future	וְיֵשׁ־תִּקְוָה לְאַחֲרִיתֵךְ
—declares God:	נְאֻם־יְיָ
Your children shall return to their country.	וְשָׁבוּ בָנִים לִגְבוּלָם:
(Jeremiah 31:15-17)	

At her son's funeral, intermingled with immense pain, Rachel Goldberg-Polin also spoke of hope, of her belief that Hersh was reunited with dead loved ones from October 7 and before. Amazingly she also spoke of *hakarat hatov*—gratitude. In her darkest moment she found the gratitude to exude thankfulness for the gift of Hersh, "the perfect son for me." Just as Jeremiah speaks words of comfort and hope in the midst of darkness, Rachel Goldberg-Polin is a resplendent exemplar of transforming trauma into growth and righteousness. Right after getting up from shivah, she recorded a message imploring the world to bring home the remaining hostages in memory of her son and the others lost alongside him.

This thread of honoring trauma's shattering darkness and yet letting it be our teacher and our motivator runs through the chapters of *The Sacred Struggle*. Our authors were called to share their struggles and those of their communities in the hope that good could come from them—comfort, wisdom, and guidance that could help ease the struggle of someone else, and even change the world for the better.

The Sacred Struggle set out to provide a usable and practical Jewish anthology to navigate and find comfort in the most difficult parts of life—the parts that are infrequently talked about and leave us feeling isolated from our usual networks. The connections formed in the midst of trauma are life-giving and irreplaceable—another patient in the waiting room, a survivor of the same disaster, a fellow grieving parent—someone who sees you and knows what you are suffering because they have stood where you stand. We hope that this book can provide a small sliver of that companionship for those who are suffering and a small window of understanding to those who are supporting others dealing with trauma. Even so, it is important to recognize that there will be readers who do not find themselves in these pages—those whose struggles are not voiced in this volume or those who went through similar experiences with vastly different reactions, feelings, and learnings. We hope this will inspire readers to share their own stories, because there are people who need to hear them. This book is your invitation to add your own wisdom to the broken and beautiful anthology of our shared and individual trauma.

Perhaps because of our intergenerational heritage of trauma, resilience, and striving for hope, Jewish tradition emphasizes the idea of *nechemta*, literally meaning "comfort" or "compassion." There is a ritual preference that we strive not to end a Torah or haftarah reading on a low or unresolved note. Instead, we break up our Torah readings so that each reading concludes with words of resolution, a *nechemta*. When we set out to compile and share these stories, we recognized the reality that not every story has a *nechemta*. Some things cannot be tied up with a nice bow or a clear resolution. It is uncomfortable to navigate unresolved trauma in a culture that stresses polite social norms and positivity. Perhaps the *nechemta* in this volume lies in navigating that tension together, across these pages, across the generations of our people, and across the relationships that we build in our darkest moments. It is okay to not be okay for as long as it takes. And yet we are still called to search, slowly and circuitously, for the *nechemta*—in whatever form it takes and whenever the time is right. May we find comfort in one another, in each other's stories, and in the stories of our people.

נַחֲמוּ נַחֲמוּ עַמִּי יֹאמַר אֱלֹהֵיכֶם:
Comfort, oh comfort My people,
Says your God.
(Isaiah 40:1)

Contributors

Rabbi Lindsey Danziger (HUC-JIR '17, MARE), is the director of campaigns at the Religious Action Center of Reform Judaism, guiding synagogues and clergy across the country in their work to organize and mobilize for justice. She is also an adjunct professor at Hebrew Union College–Jewish Institute of Religion, where she teaches community organizing. Rabbi Danziger resides in Nashville, Tennessee, with her husband, Rabbi Michael Danziger, and their three children, Ben, Aviva, and Noa.

Rabbi Benjamin David is the senior rabbi of Reform Congregation Keneseth Israel in Elkins Park, Pennsylvania. He is a teacher of Talmud, lover of Israel, and avid runner, having completed twenty-three marathons. He is married to Lisa Bieber David, the executive director of Camp Harlam. They are the parents of Noa, Elijah, and Samuel.

Rabbi Robyn Ashworth-Steen is a British progressive rabbi who is currently pursuing justice through her academic work, both in writing and teaching. Before rabbinic ordination, Rabbi Robyn was a human rights lawyer. Rabbi Robyn seeks to contribute to anti-oppressive theo/alogies and community spaces.

Rabbi Elizabeth Bahar, MAHL, who currently serves as the spiritual leader of Temple Beth Israel in Macon, Georgia, is a published author whose recent works include chapters in *The Sacred Earth: Jewish Perspectives on Our Planet* (CCAR Press, 2023) and *Prophetic Voices Renewing and Reimagining Haftarah* (CCAR Press, 2023) Beyond her congregational leadership, which has earned her multiple Rabbi Jeffrey L. Ballon Interfaith Leadership Awards, she combines her pastoral expertise with academia as an adjunct professor of Hebrew Bible at Mercer University's College of Professional Advancement. *The Forward* recognized Rabbi Bahar as one of "America's 33 Most Inspirational Rabbis" in 2015; she continues to bridge interfaith relationships while advancing Jewish education and community engagement.

Rabbi Leah Cohen Tenenbaum, DMin, BCC-PCHAC, serves as the inpatient palliative care chaplain at Yale New Haven Hospital. She is a graduate of HUC-JIR (Cincinnati '00), a faculty member of FASPE (Fellowships at Auschwitz for the Study of Professional Ethics), and has served on the CCAR Board of Trustees, the CCAR National Ethics Taskforce, and currently on the CCAR Press Council. Coeditor with Rabbi Douglas Kohn of the forthcoming book *Striving to Be Human: Jewish Perspectives on Twenty-First Century Challenges* (CCAR Press), she frequently teaches and presents on spirituality, serious illness, and medical ethics.

Rabbi Charlie Cytron-Walker is the rabbi at Temple Emanuel in Winston-Salem, North Carolina and formerly served as the rabbi of Congregation Beth Israel in Colleyville, Texas. Since "The Incident," Rabbi Charlie has spoken at the White House, testified before Congress, and has been published in numerous news sources.

Rabbi Harry K. Danziger is rabbi emeritus of Temple Israel, Memphis, where he served from 1964 until his retirement in 2000. He is past president of the Central Conference of American Rabbis and past board chair of the Metropolitan Inter-Faith Association. He was on the faculty of Rhodes College for thirty years and, after retirement, served as visiting rabbi of Congregation B'nai Israel, Cleveland, Mississippi, for two decades.

Rabbi Denise L. Eger is a past president of the Central Conference of American Rabbis. She is an executive and leadership coach for clergy and nonprofit executives. She is founding rabbi emerita of Congregation Kol Ami in West Hollywood, California and the author of *Mishkan Ga'avah: Where Pride Dwells, A Celebration of LGBTQ Jewish Life and Ritual* (CCAR Press, 2020) and *7 Principles for Living Bravely: Ageless Wisdom and Comforting Faith for Weathering Life's Most Difficult Times* (TGK Press, 2023).

Deborah L. Greene is a Jewish educator, blogger, and activist. She's written extensively about suicide loss and traumatic grief on her blog, *ReflectingOutLoud.net*, as well as publications like *The Forward, Reform Judaism.org, The Mighty,* and *The Year of Mourning: A Jewish Journey* (CCAR

Press, 2023). She is part of the Congregation Har HaShem community in Boulder, Colorado.

Rabbi Daniel Gropper, DD, has served as spiritual leader of Community Synagogue of Rye—a caring Jewish community that adds meaning and purpose to your life—since 2003. Prior to that he served congregations in Lexington, Massachusetts, Scarsdale, New York, South Lake Tahoe, California, and Santa Monica, California. He holds an MAJE and MAHL from HUC-JIR along with rabbinic ordination (NY '98) and has competed in numerous bike races and triathlons.

Rabbi Jen Gubitz (she/her) is a rabbi at Temple Shalom of Newton, Massachusetts and the founder of Modern Jewish Couples. A graduate of Indiana University's Borns Jewish Studies program, Jen was ordained from HUC-JIR (NY) in 2012. She is the co-host of the *OMfG Podcast: Jewish Wisdom for Unprecedented Times* and her writing appears in the *Los Angeles Times, Romper, Boston Globe, OnBeing, Jewish Daily Forward*, and *Lilith Magazine*. She lives in Boston with her husband and offers tremendous gratitude to the God of Science and Stardust for their son, Ori Shir. Learn more at www.jengubitz.com.

Rabbi Debra R. Hachen followed in the footsteps of her father and great-grandfather when she was ordained in 1980 by Hebrew Union College–Jewish Institute of Religion. She is the founding rabbi and rabbi emerita of Congregation B'nai Shalom in Westborough, Massachusetts, and also served two synagogues in New Jersey. While in rabbinic school she met and married her husband, Peter Weinrobe, a former regional youth advisor for National Federation of Temple Youth in Southern California. They have three children and six grandchildren. After thirty-seven years in the rabbinate, Rabbi Hachen took early retirement to relocate near family in California to be a full-time wife and caregiver to her husband.

Rabbi Lawrence A. Hoffman, PhD, is the Barbara Friedman Professor Emeritus of Liturgy, Worship, and Ritual at the Hebrew Union College–Jewish Institute of Religion in New York, where he served for over half a century. In 1994, he co-founded "Synagogue 2000" a trans-denominational project to envision the ideal synagogue "as moral and spiritual center" for the twenty-first century. He founded, and still directs, the Bonnie Tisch Initiative for Jewish Excellence, a program that offers curricular enrichment to promising rabbinic and cantorial students. He has authored or edited fifty books; and his current thinking can be followed in a series of "Open Letters to My Students" which appear on his blog, *Life and a Little Liturgy*.

Rabbi David N. Jaffe was born in Louisville, Kentucky and is currently serving as co-rabbi of Temple Kol Tikvah in Davidson, North Carolina with his wife, Rabbi Becca Diamond. Rabbi Jaffe holds a bachelor of arts in music from Centre College (2012), a master of music in trumpet performance from the University of Louisville (2014), and rabbinic ordination from the Cincinnati campus of HUC-JIR (2022). Rabbi Jaffe has two beautiful boxer dogs, Ginny and Hermione.

Rabbi Debra Kassoff is a regional organizer for Working Together Mississippi and, for the last fifteen years, has served as spiritual leader of her former student pulpit, Hebrew Union Congregation in Greenville, Mississippi. She has spent most of her rabbinate in Mississippi, joining the Institute of Southern Jewish Life in Jackson as its first director of rabbinic services following her ordination in 2003 (HUC-JIR, Cincinnati). Rabbi Kassoff finds sustenance and joy in the work of building communities that embrace and transcend difference, and in sharing life with her husband Alec, their two amazing children, and beloved friends in Jackson, Mississippi.

Rabbi Paul Kipnes (NY '92) is spiritual leader of Congregation Or Ami, Calabasas, California. He is author of *The Secret Life of the Mourner: A Poetic Journey Through a Year of Mourning* (lulu.com), and coauthor with his wife Michelle November of *Jewish Spiritual Parenting: Wisdom, Activities, Rituals and Prayers for Raising Children with Spiritual Balance and Emotional Wholeness*. He inspires others at paulkipnes.com.

Adriane Leveen, PhD, is senior lecturer emeritus in Hebrew Bible at Hebrew Union College–Jewish Institute of Religion. She has published two books, *Memory and Tradition in the Book of Numbers* (2008) and *Biblical Narratives of Israelites and Their Neighbors: Strangers at the Gate* (2017).

She has published numerous articles and is currently at work on popular responses to the Book of Job.

Rabbi Serge A. Lippe is a graduate of the Bronx High School of Science, the College of the University of Chicago, and was ordained at HUC-JIR, New York, in 1991. He served as the associate rabbi of Temple Solel in Paradise Valley, Arizona. He has guided the Brooklyn Heights Synagogue as its spiritual leader for the last twenty-seven years. He is the editor *of Birkon Artzi: Blessings and Meditations for Travelers to Israel* (CCAR Press, 2012).

Rabbi Robert (Bob) H. Loewy (HUC-JIR, NY '77) is the rabbi emeritus of Congregation Gates of Prayer in Metairie, Louisiana, a synagogue he served from 1984–2018. Beyond the congregation, his rabbinate includes the Greater New Orleans Jewish and interfaith community, along with a variety of positions with the CCAR and Reform Movement. He is married to Lynn (Rosenfeld) Loewy, is blessed with four children, and is "Papa" to six grandchildren.

Rabbi Dalia Marx, PhD, a tenth-generation Jerusalemite, is the Rabbi Aaron D. Panken Professor of Liturgy at Hebrew Union College–Jewish Institute of Religion in Jerusalem. She is the author of several books, including *From Time to Time: Journeys in the Jewish Calendar* (CCAR Press, 2024), *A Feminist Commentary on the Babylonian Talmud: Tractates Tamid, Middot, and Qinnim* (Mohr Siebeck, 2013), and the coeditor of several others, including *T'filat HaAdam*, the Israeli Reform prayer book (MARAM, 2020). Rabbi Marx and her husband Roly Zylbersztein, PhD, live in Jerusalem; they have three children.

Rabbah Rona Matlow, DMin (ze/hir) is an elder disabled veteran, genderpunk non-binary transgender woman rabbi and scholar. Hir research is in the areas of Bible and diversity. Ze has published many anthology chapters, a journal article, web entries, and a book.

Rabbi Joel Mosbacher is the senior rabbi of Temple Shaaray Tefila in New York, having served congregations in Mahwah, New Jersey and Atlanta, Georgia. He has been a leader in community organizing with the Industrial Areas Foundation since 2005. He and his wife Elyssa are the proud parents of Ari and Lili.

Rabbi Robert A. Nosanchuk serves as inaugural senior rabbi and Will & Jan Sukenik Chair in Rabbinics of Congregation Mishkan Or in Cleveland, Ohio. He is entirely in love with his spouse Joanie Berger, proud as one can be of their two young adult children, and alive today due to the medical team at Cleveland Clinic who saved him from a fast-growing Stage IV metastatic cancer. He is now in remission for the first time in five years, a cancer survivor intent to realize a comeback in mental and physical health in the "bonus time" that lies ahead.

Rabbi Rex D. Perlmeter, LSW, (HUC-JIR, '85) served as spiritual leader of Temple Israel of Greater Miami (1985–1996) and Baltimore Hebrew Congregation (1996–2008), before joining the staff at the Union for Reform Judaism for five years. He founded the Jewish Wellness Center of North Jersey, trained as a Jewish Mindfulness Meditation teacher and a spiritual director, and received his master of social work from New York University in May, 2016. He was the CCAR's special advisor for member support and counseling from 2014–2023, currently serves as an adjunct faculty member at HUC-JIR, and maintains a small private practice in spiritual direction and clinical therapy.

Rabbi Karen Glazer Perolman is the senior associate rabbi at Temple B'nai Jeshurun in Short Hills, New Jersey, the congregation she has served since 2008. While in rabbinical school at the Hebrew Union College–Jewish Institute of Religion in New York, her theology was nurtured through her work serving as a teaching assistant to theologian Rabbi Eugene B. Borowitz, PhD, *z"l*. Her writings have been published online and in four CCAR Press publications: *The Sacred Table: Creating a Jewish Food Ethic* (2011), *Moral Resistance and Spiritual Authority: Our Jewish Obligation to Social Justice* (2019), *The Sacred Encounter: Jewish Perspectives on Sexuality* (2014), and *Mishkan Ga'avah: Where Pride Dwells* (2020).

Rabbi Iah Pillsbury (she/they) received her undergraduate degree from the University of Chicago, and was ordained by Hebrew Union College–Jewish Institute of Religion in Cincinnati. They currently serve a URJ congregation in Colorado Springs, Colorado where she enjoys spending her free time with her wife and children.

Rabbi Daniel A. Roberts (DD, DMin, FT, USN) is rabbi emeritus of Temple Emanu El, Cleveland, Ohio, where he served for over thirty-five years. He is also a Fellow in Thanatology as certified by the Association of Death Education and Counseling and has done extensive work on bereavement and mourning. Rabbi Roberts is the author of four books including *Clergy Retirement: Every Ending a New Beginning* (Wipf & Stock, 2017). Presently, Rabbi Roberts serves a monthly congregation in Rapid City, South Dakota, and lives in Denver, Colorado.

Yolanda Savage-Narva (she/her) is the vice president of Racial Equity, Diversity, and Inclusion (REDI) and Communities of Belonging for the Union for Reform Judaism. For more than twenty years, Yolanda collaborated with Tribal governments to strengthen public health systems, promoted pedestrian safety and advocacy, coined the phrase, "Walking is a civil right," and advanced health equity in states and territories. Most recently, Yolanda was the executive director with Operation Understanding DC, a nonprofit organization dedicated to promoting understanding, cooperation, and respect while fighting to eradicate racism, antisemitism, and all forms of discrimination. Yolanda is also on the boards of the American Jewish World Services, the Capital Jewish Museum, Leading Edge, the Federation of Greater Washington, and the historic Sixth and I Synagogue in Washington, DC. Yolanda is also a member of Delta Sigma Theta Sorority, an international Black sorority dedicated to community service and education.

Rabbi Adrienne Pollock Scott was ordained from HUC-JIR in 2004. Since 2005, she has served at Congregation Beth Israel in Houston, Texas, and now holds the position of senior associate rabbi. Rabbi Scott is passionate about pastoral care and guiding her congregants to fulfill their own spiritual quests through ritual, prayer, and music. Rabbi Scott is married to David, RJE, and they are the proud parents of Beryt and Ezra.

After serving congregations in Atlanta, Georgia, and Alexandria, Viriginia, **Rabbi David Spinrad** returned home in 2025 to his Bay Area roots to serve Beth Chaim Congregation in Danville, California. He is a former member of the CCAR's Board of Trustees, Convention

Planning Committee, and served as chairperson of the Justice, Peace, and Civil Liberties Committee. Additionally, David authored "Digging Isaac's Third Well: Water and Systemic Racism," a chapter on *Parashat Tol'dot* in *The Social Justice Torah Commentary* (CCAR Press, 2021). An avid sports card collector, for fun he hosts "The Rated Rabbi Sports Card Podcast."

Rabbi Shira Stern was ordained as a rabbi from Hebrew Union College–Jewish Institute of Religion in 1983 and earned her Doctor of Ministry there in 2004. She has served in two pulpits in New Jersey and has been a hospital and hospice chaplain as well. She was the director of the Jewish Institute for Pastoral Care, part of the HealthCare Chaplaincy, providing programs students, chaplains and clergy in the field. She was also a past-president of the National Association of Jewish Chaplains. She currently serves the ARC as co-lead for Disaster Spiritual Care (DSC) in Massachusetts and Northern New England and is the DSC division advisor for the Northeast region. She is a board certified chaplain and a board certified pastoral counselor in private practice, providing individual and family therapy.

Rabbi Melissa Zalkin Stollman is currently a freelance rabbi serving multiple congregations as a marketing consultant while also serving unaffiliated Jews for life cycle events. Rabbi Stollman has a master in social work from Boston University and rabbinic ordination and a master in religious education from the Hebrew Union College–Jewish Institute of Religion. In her free time, Rabbi Stollman enjoys teaching mat-based Pilates and Barre, all things digital media, playing mahjongg, singing and strumming her guitar, and spending time with her husband and their family.

Betsy Stone, PhD, tackles some of the most difficult issues facing individuals, families, and organizations today: developing character, dealing with stress and anxiety, facing trauma and its aftermath. Her optimism, critical thinking, and hopeful approach help people find ways to change and grow. She invites discussion and ideas, and is skilled at creating opportunities for your organization to tackle complex ideas. As an experienced psychologist, she understands how people change and what impedes growth. Whether in workshops, webinars, lectures, or scholar-in-residence experiences, Dr. Stone helps people figure out what they are ready to learn, and then teaches it.

Rabbi Susan B. Stone was ordained at the Cincinnati campus of HUC-JIR in 1983. She is currently director of spiritual care at Hillcrest Hospital, a Cleveland Clinic Hospital. She is married to Wayne Easthon and, blessedly, their family keeps growing.

Rabbi Aaron A. Stucker-Rozovsky has been humbled to serve the wonderful folks of Beth El Congregation in Winchester, Virginia since 2020 with the love and support of his incredible wife, Dr. Eliza Stucker-Rozovsky. He is a graduate of Providence College, Central Connecticut State University, and Hebrew Union College–Jewish Institute of Religion. In addition to being blessed with a pulpit, Rabbi Stucker-Rozovsky proudly serves our beloved country as an Army Reserve chaplain with nineteen years in uniform, including several overseas deployments in support of the Global War on Terror.

Rabbi Susan Talve is the founding rabbi and rabbi emerita of Central Reform Congregation, the only synagogue within the city limits of St. Louis, Missouri. She is also the founder of the Ashrei Foundation, an organization dedicated to disrupting cycles of poverty and lifting up the marginalized and oppressed. She is a grateful daughter, wife, mother, and grandmother, and works every day to make her late daughter Adina, proud.

Rabbi Ariel Tovlev, MAJE (he/they) is a poet and educator who serves as the spiritual leader of Kehila Chadasha in the Maryland suburbs of DC. Among the first trans rabbis ordained by HUC-JIR, he intimately knows the pain of having to forge new pathways and is passionate about creating spaces of belonging for marginalized Jews. Their writing has been featured in other CCAR Press titles, including *Prophetic Voices, The First Fifty Years*, and *Mishkan Ga'avah: Where Pride Dwells*.

Rabbi Ari Vernon was ordained at the Jewish Theological Seminary in 2004. He serves as the Judaic Studies department chair at The Emery/Weiner School in Houston, Texas, where he has been a member of the faculty for over fifteen years. In addition, Rabbi Vernon serves Congregation Shalom Rav in Austin, Texas, and is the cantorial soloist at Temple Sinai in Houston. A passionate lover of Israel, he enjoys yoga, Disney, playing the guitar, and spending time with his three amazing children.

Rabbi Annie Villarreal-Belford, PsyD (she, her), a native of El Paso, Texas, received a bachelor of arts in creative writing from the University of Judaism (*summa cum laude*), a master in Hebrew letters, and rabbinic ordination from Hebrew Union College–Jewish Institute of Religion, and a PsyD in pastoral logotherapy from Graduate Theological Seminary. She was the first full-time female solo rabbi in Houston, serving Temple Sinai from 2009–2022, and currently works as Editor at CCAR Press. In her free time, she enjoys reading, art journaling, visiting National Parks, and loves nothing more than soaking up life with her wife and three children.

Rabbi Dvora Weisberg, PhD is the Rabbi Aaron D. Panken Professor of Rabbinics on the Los Angeles campus of Hebrew Union College–Jewish Institute of Religion. Rabbi Weisberg's research focuses on gender and the family in the Babylonian Talmud. She is a member of the CCAR Responsa Committee.

Rabbi Marina Yergin is the associate rabbi at Temple Beth-El in San Antonio, Texas, where she has been serving since ordination from Hebrew Union College–Jewish Institute of Religion in Cincinnati in 2015. She previously wrote a chapter in *The Social Justice Torah Commentary* (CCAR Press, 2021) and has been published on Ritualwell.org. Since 2021, she has been diligently working on the Reform Movement's ethical misconduct processes, particularly with the Union for Reform Judaism. In this capacity, she found herself representing survivors and presenting the restorative justice work during the Safety, Respect, and Equity Conference in 2024 with Rabbi Mary Zamore, Rabbi Rick Jacobs, Dr. Alissa Ackerman, and Dr. Guila Benchimol.

Rabbi Wendy Zierler, PhD, is the Sigmund Falk Professor of Modern Jewish Literature and Feminist Studies at HUC-JIR in New York. A literary historian and fiction writer, Rabbi Zierler has focused on, among other things, questions of gender in modern Hebrew fiction and poetry.

Her book, *Movies and Midrash: Popular Film and Jewish Religious Conversation* (SUNY Press) was a finalist for the 2017 National Jewish Book Award. Her newest book, *Going Out with Knots: My Two Kaddish Years with Hebrew Poetry*, is forthcoming in 2025 from the Jewish Publication Society / University of Nebraska Press. Rabbi Zierler received her PhD from Princeton University, her MFA in fiction writing from Sarah Lawrence College, and rabbinic ordination from Yeshivat Maharat.

www.ingramcontent.com/pod-product-compliance
Lightning Source LLC
Chambersburg PA
CBHW032316210326
41518CB00040B/1011